UNDERSTANDING CANCER

a Consumer Publication

Consumers' Association
publishers of **Which?**
14 Buckingham Street
London WC2N 6DS

Throughout this book

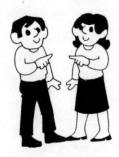

for 'he' read 'he or she'

CONTENTS

FOREWORD

We all have to die some time but we hope to reach a ripe old age before this happens. We certainly do not want to have a serious illness that could kill us when we are younger. Cancer has this reputation, but in some ways it is exaggerated. In the first place, cancer is usually a disease of older people, and in the second place it is not the commonest cause of death. Nearly twice as many people die of heart attacks than of cancer. Only about one-fifth of the population die of cancer. That is bad enough, but it puts cancer into perspective.

Just as people try to prevent heart disease, by exercise and diet, so we could take steps to reduce our chances of getting cancer, if we really wanted to. People become very concerned about the small numbers of extra cancers caused by radiation, but the real epidemic is in lung cancer which could largely be avoided if people gave up cigarettes.

Cancer researchers are constantly pressed by the media for a dramatic 'breakthrough'. There are no instant or miracle cures, but we are working on the problem and it must be remembered that there has been tremendous progress already this century, from curing less than 5% of all cancers in 1900 to over 50% in 1985. Since lung cancers are so difficult to cure, that average would rise very rapidly if the smokers could be persuaded to stop.

There is plenty left to do and this book helps to show the way. It puts the subject into perspective and shows ordinary people what they can do, to avoid the known causes, to recognise the early signs of cancer and to seek treatment at that stage, when it is most effective, and to avoid unproven remedies. But since not all cancers can be cured, we need to know that people can live in reasonable comfort with cancer, just as they can with high blood pressure and other incurable diseases. If there is pain, then it can be relieved; and so can most of the other problems if the right people are looking after things. We all have to die some time but in the 1980s the word cancer need not mean fear and despair.

Professor A H W Nias

Richard Dimbleby Department of Cancer Research,
United Medical and Dental Schools, St Thomas' Hospital, London

THE NATURE OF CANCER

The term cancer is applied to a wide range of diseases that have several attributes in common

○ a disorganised cell growth
○ ability to spread
○ cellular changes

but have different origins, manifest themselves in different ways and call for different methods of treatment.

These diseases occur in individuals of all ages in communities throughout the world, but certain cancers are particularly associated with certain age groups or areas: some occur most frequently in children, some in old people, and others are more commonly found in the developed countries than the under-developed.

disorganised cell growth

All cancers are the result of the uncontrolled over-production of some particular cells. Normally, worn-out cells are replaced by a process of cell division. But if new cells are produced in excess of what is needed for replacement, there occurs a build-up of tissue. When this forms a mass or tumour, it may cause symptoms such as swelling, the obstruction of a hollow organ, and sometimes, but by no means always, pain.

Not all tumours resulting from disorganised growth are malignant, that is, cancerous: some are benign – for example, a wart is a benign (that is, not cancerous) tumour.

Uncontrolled reproduction of cells, unless compensated for by an equally large number of cell deaths, can in a few generations of cells produce thousands of cells from a single cell source. Each cell division doubles the number of cells, and represents one generation. It is not that cancer cells always reproduce much faster than normal cells, but rather that they die off more slowly.

Forty doublings can produce 10^{12} cells (a million million), a tumour of over one kilogram, which would usually be lethal. Most human cancers are probably not detectable before they are considerably advanced along this road: 10^6 cells (twenty doublings) are not detectable; 10^9 cells (thirty doublings) are just detectable as one gram of tumour, approximately one cubic centimetre, the size of a small sugar cube.

Cancers arising in different tissues have very different growth rates; this is due partly to the fact that each kind of cell has its own rate of multiplication, and partly to the varying ability of cancer cells to derive adequate nutrients and oxygen supplies. This factor in turn depends on the cancer's blood supply, which also influences the rate at which cancer cells die.

ability to spread
Cancer cells infiltrate or invade the surrounding normal tissues. Benign tumours, on the other hand, merely grow locally, usually enclosed within a capsule; they can eventually compress the adjacent tissues, sometimes painfully or even dangerously, but without invading them.

distant spread
Metastasis (*meta* is greek for beyond) is really an extension of spreading. Cancer cells are able to gain access to the blood circulation, and also to the lymphatic system (whose function is to drain the tissues and combat infection). They insinuate themselves between the cells which line the blood vessels or lymphatic vessels. By these conduits, the cancer cells are carried to other organs, where they lodge to form secondary tumours, or metastases, far from the tissues or organs where the cancer originated.

cellular changes
Cancer cells undergo changes which make them different from normal tissue. Such differences may not be at all obvious: individual cancer cells may look very similar to normal cells, even under a high magnification microscope, but they behave differently.

the normal cell

The cell is the basic unit from which all the tissues of the body are built up: there are a number of cell types, defined according to the function of each organ. The cell is a microscopic particle of protoplasm – the material from which the body is built up, consisting mainly of proteins. Each cell is separated from other cells by a thin wall or membrane, and contains a nucleus which controls it. That part of the cell which is neither membrane nor nucleus is called cytoplasm.

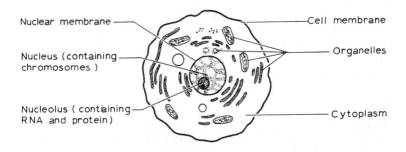

Nuclear membrane ————— ————— Cell membrane

Nucleus (containing ————— ————— Organelles
chromosomes)

Nucleolus (containing ————— ————— Cytoplasm
RNA and protein)

cell membrane: this controls the passage of nutrients in and out of the cell.

cell cytoplasm: the cell obtains its energy from the combustion of nutrients, which takes place in the cytoplasm in organelles, structures which carry out different functions. Enzymes, essential proteins which activate all chemical reactions in the cell, are also formed in the organelles.

nucleus: this is separated from the cytoplasm by a membrane of its own. It contains information about all of the cell's individual characteristics, packaged as a coded message in structures called chromosomes, which contain many small links, called genes. Each of these contains a section of DNA (deoxyribonucleic acid), the material of inheritance, together with RNA (ribonucleic acid), which acts as a pattern or template for the production of new proteins. In effect, a cell's genes are a set of instructions, telling the cell how and in what order to go about the process of replicating itself. Thus, when a cell reproduces itself by a process of division (called mitosis), the daughter cells will be exact replicas of the parent.

Techniques for reading the DNA codes are being widely developed by biologists, and will, it is hoped, eventually make it possible to understand what causes the normal cell to become cancerous.

cancer cells
It is suspected that the development of cancer cells from normal cells is essentially the result of some alteration in the cellular DNA. The effects are uncontrolled reproduction, infiltration and distant spread.

Sometimes cancer cells can be recognised because they contain a relative deficiency or excess of certain enzymes.

differentiated and undifferentiated cancers
When cancer cells look broadly similar to those of the tissue in which they grew, they are said to be 'well differentiated'. In some cases, however, they exhibit very different appearances. When the cancer cells are bizarrely unlike the cells of the tissue in which they are found, so that there is uncertainty whether they originated there, the cancer is said to be 'poorly differentiated' (or *anaplastic* from the greek *ana* = backwards, *plassein* = to form).

The reason for this apparently paradoxical usage is this: in the very early stages of an embryo's growth, immediately after conception, its cells are all of one kind, that is, undifferentiated. As the embryo grows, the cells develop in different ways and acquire specialised functions, becoming the various tissues and organs: they become differentiated. Poorly differentiated or anaplastic cancers look unlike the specialised tissue in which they grow, because the cancer cells have lost their specialised appearance, and look more like the unspecialised sort, not recognisable as arising from any one particular organ.

Poorly differentiated cancers usually grow much faster and metastasise more easily than the well differentiated kind, which tend to grow more slowly, and spread less easily. A tumour may contain both poorly differentiated and well differentiated cells.

how cancers are classified

Medical terminology assigns cancers to broad subdivisions, according to the body tissues in which they originate: thus

carcinoma is used for cancer of the epithelial tissues, such as skin, or stomach lining;

sarcoma is cancer of bone, connective tissues, such as sinews, muscles;

leukaemias are related to the white blood cells, *lymphomas* to the lymphatic system.

The greek suffix *-oma* is used when there is a tumour or swelling. Cancers are generally described as malignant tumours or malignant neoplasms (greek, *neo* = new; *plasma* = form). The study of such tumours is now generally known as oncology.

secondary cancer

A cancer which has spread (metastasised) and is growing in a tissue distant from its origin is called a secondary cancer.

Virtually any organ can be invaded by secondary cancers. The commonest sites are the lymph glands, lungs, bone, liver and brain. This is partly due to the high rate of blood or lymph flow through these organs, which are thus constantly exposed to travelling cancer cells. When first signs of illness are observed, secondary cancers may or may not already be present: it depends on the site where the primary cancer started, the degree of differentiation and the cell type of the cancer. Some primary cancers produce only minor symptoms, or none at all, at the original site, and so go unremarked, until symptoms arise which are caused by the secondary cancers – by which time the disease could be too widespread for effective treatment.

lymph nodes (lymph glands)

The lymphatic system is the drainage system of the tissues: it is a network of vessels called lymphatics, similar to blood vessels, covering all the organs (except the nervous system). They drain lymph, a yellowish watery fluid, derived from the blood circulation, out of the infinitesimally small spaces between the cells. At intervals on the lymph network, strategically placed to cover certain regions or organs, there occur lymph nodes or lymph glands which act as filtering stations for these regions. They are the source of immune defence cells and antibodies which destroy any bacteria in the lymph before it is drained back into the blood circulation.

These nodes often swell up and become tender when there is infection near them. In the vast majority of cases, swollen neck or groin nodes do not mean cancer, but usually point to local infection.

This is the beneficial aspect of the lymph nodes. However, the lymphatic network also helps cancers to spread, by acting as their transport system. The lymph nodes are sites where secondary cancers are often found. Because the lymphatics from certain organs drain into particular groups of lymph nodes, the secondary cancers give a clue about where the malignancy started.

Lymph node sites of **secondary cancers**	Likely sites of **primary cancers**
Cervical (neck)	lungs, nose, throat, tongue, breast, gastro-intestinal tract (stomach, liver, intestines, etc.) skin
Axillary (armpit)	breast, skin, arm (bone in)
Mediastinal (chest between the lungs)	lungs, testes
Abdominal (belly)	genito-urinary system (bladder, bowels, sex organs, etc.), gastro-intestinal tract
Inguinal (groin)	skin, vulva, legs (bone in)

Primary lymph node cancers (lymphomas) such as Hodgkin's disease can arise in or spread to any or all of the other lymph nodes.

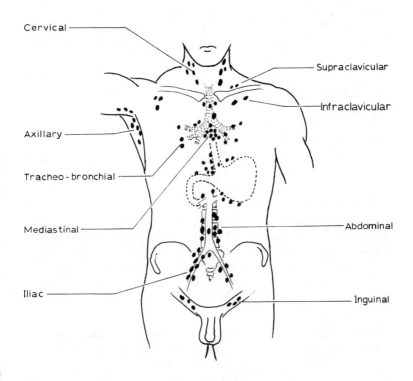

The main groups of lymph nodes in the body.

THE CAUSES OF CANCER

Cancer is considered to be not one disease but many: it is possible that the various types of the disease have different causes, or a number of causes and that various different events have to happen to cause cancer. In the case of some cancers, the cause is pretty well established: for instance, the connection between smoking and lung cancer is no longer seriously questioned. But there may be some other factors involved, because not everybody who smokes gets cancer.

One way of shedding light on more obscure causes of some cancers is through epidemiological research.

Cancer occurs world-wide, but most forms are more common in some communities than in others. A study of the differences between countries (or communities) in the incidence of some cancers often gives some ideas of possible causes. The science of studying the patterns of the disease in populations is called epidemiology. It has made great contributions towards our understanding of cancer and, in fact, the smoking–lung cancer link was arrived at mainly through epidemiological research.

Epidemiologists can study cancer from two aspects: the incidence of disease, which records how many new cases of a particular cancer are reported in a population during a stated period of time (usually a year); and the mortality, which records how many people die of this type of cancer in the same period. In the UK, these data are collated by the Office of Population Censuses and surveys with the help of several cancer registries which rely on hospital notification and death certification.

Such research has shown that the incidence of most cancers can very enormously not only between countries, but also between different communities within one country and at different times within the same community.

Studies have shown that differences in cancer incidence occur even between different religious sects as well as between different socio-economic and racial groups. The differences are more likely to be based on the abstention from practices such as smoking, than on the varieties of belief in God.

The total incidence of cancer of all types does not vary greatly between countries, but the incidence of particular types of cancer varies considerably, and any cancer that is frequent in one community is usually rare in at least one other community. Epidemiological studies have demonstrated differences in cancer incidence between different countries which seem to be related to certain important factors, such as age, heredity and environment.

age and the occurrence of cancer
Although some forms of cancer can occur at any age, about 50% of all cancers occur in people over the age of 55. Most cancers are rare in the young and become progressively more frequent as age advances, especially from the middle fifties onwards. This is especially true of the commonest cancers of western society, namely lung, breast, prostate, bowel, bladder cancers. However, cancers can (and do) develop in any of the body's organs and tissues at any age.

An ageing population, such as that of Great Britain, shows an increase in cancer incidence.

The age effect apart, some specific cancers are generally on the increase, for example, cancer of the colon and malignant melanoma; other cancers are becoming less common, for example, cancer of the stomach and of the oesophagus.

heredity v. environment
These are two major factors. It is often difficult to distinguish between the effects of heredity and of environment, because just as one inherits one's parents' and grandparents' genes, so one also generally inherits their environment. Epidemiological studies are thus specially interested in migrant populations which essentially succeed in maintaining their genetic characteristics in a new country. Such studies have pointed to the environment as the likeliest cause of variations.

For instance, cancer incidences in Japan and in the USA are very different, yet Japanese inhabitants of Hawaii and mainland USA tend to show cancer rates similar to those of native Americans of mainly European origin. Particularly striking is the increase in bowel cancer and the fall in stomach cancer.

Coronary heart disease shows analogous changes: Japanese in Japan have a much lower rate of this disease than Americans, but Japanese migrants to the USA within a couple of generations come to equal the American rate. In that instance, the underlying cause is thought to be dietary, the change from the Japanese diet, low in dairy products and animal fats, to the American diet, high in both. There are indications that the higher rate of bowel and breast cancer among Japanese migrants and the lower rate of stomach cancer are similarly determined.

genetic predisposition

Certain cancers tend to 'run' in families, for example, retinoblastoma, a cancer of the eye. Breast cancer occurs in first-degree female relatives (sister, daughter) of women with the disease approximately twice as frequently as the average for the female population. This does not necessarily mean that specific genetic factors are involved: the epidemiological data strongly suggest that environmental factors have a big part to play. That women with breast cancer share some genetic predisposition to the disease, remains a possibility.

Occasionally, inherited diseases predispose to specific cancers – for example, familial polyposis coli, a condition in which polyps grow in the colon, harmless in themselves but predisposing to cancer of the bowel.

It is likely that in many cases both genetic and environmental factors are important, and that genetic factors characterise a sub-group of the population at greater risk of the cancer, and that environmental factors determine the proportion of that sub-group who actually get the cancer (and so determine the overall risk in a population). It is possible that genetic factors cause variations in sensitivity to environmental factors.

environmental causes of cancer

The fact that the incidence of cancer in western society rises with age, the peak period for cancer risk being late middle age onwards, suggests that carcinogenesis (the formation of a cancer) may in many cases take place after years, even decades of exposure. Lung cancer resulting from smoking may be an example of this. This effect cannot be readily imitated in a laboratory. It is very difficult to design laboratory experiments that offer the exact equivalent of human exposure to carcinogens (substances which have a tendency to cause cancer).

Even when carcinogenesis occurs comparatively promptly after exposure, it may not be simple to associate this effect, when produced in a laboratory, with what actually happens in human beings. There are many substances that have been shown to affect chromosomal DNA in the laboratory: such change (or mutation) predisposes to abnormal changes in cells and to the formation of cancer. However, describing what happens to the DNA in the cells of rodents, or 'cell lines' in tissue culture in the laboratory, is not the same as being able to tell what will happen in man.

Epidemiological evidence has, however, convincingly associated certain environmental factors with the risk of specific cancers. For example, skin cancers in light-skinned people are associated with an excessive exposure to the ultraviolet (UV) radiation in sunlight. Exposure to asbestos dust causes mesothelioma (a cancer of the membrane lining the chest cavity, the lungs and the intestines); excessive X-ray exposure has been shown to cause leukaemia and other cancers.

Emissions from radioactive substances have been known to be carcinogenic since their effect was identified in uranium miners in Germany, and in pioneering physicists such as some of Marie Curie's co-workers who died of leukaemia.

life style and cancer

Epidemiologists do not start by examining a number of pollutants and then look for corresponding diseases. Rather, they look at patterns of disease and then try to determine what may have produced them.

cigarette smoking

Cigarette smoking is outstandingly associated with an increased risk of cancer of the lung, throat, mouth, lip, larynx and oesophagus. What is more, because some of the components of cigarette smoke are absorbed through the lungs into the bloodstream, smoking probably increases the risk of cancer in the pancreas and bladder and possibly the kidneys.

Because the effects of smoking often do not come to light until after many years of tobacco use, there was an enormous increase in the lung cancer death rate in men, twenty to forty years after the first world war, a period during which cigarette smoking in young men increased markedly. However, there is now a definite decline in lung cancer amongst men under 60, and this may be due both to a change to low-tar cigarettes and to a reduction in the amount smoked.

One can judge the magnitude of the effect of cigarette smoking by examining the cancer incidence in smokers and in non-smokers. If the whole population of the UK were non-smokers, the annual total of lung cancer deaths would be about 3,500. However, the actual total of such deaths is nearly 40,000 a year, and the difference of more than 35,000 deaths between these totals can be ascribed to smoking tobacco. Similarly with cancers of the upper digestive tract, the bladder and the pancreas: the comparison of the incidence of these in smokers and non-smokers reveals a further 11,000 deaths which can be put down to smoking. The total number of deaths from cancer due to smoking accounts for nearly a third of all cancer deaths.

Cigarette smoking is undoubtedly the major contributor to lung cancer, but is it the only contributor? Not all smokers actually get lung cancer: only about 10 per cent of them. One person in eight who gets lung cancer is a non-smoker. Country dwellers tend to have a lower incidence of lung cancer than people in towns. In towns, people working in some jobs – foundries, for example – have higher risks than others. All this suggests that there are also other factors at work, as well as smoking.

pipe and cigar smoking
The risk of contracting lung cancer is very much smaller for people who smoke pipes and cigars, probably because they inhale less of the smoke. However, people who switch from cigarettes to pipes or cigars may not get much benefit, as they tend to carry over their habit of inhaling. Moreover, the risk of cancer of the mouth, oesophagus (gullet) and larynx (voice-box) is much the same for all types of smokers.

alcohol
Pure alcohol (ethanol) has not been found to induce cancer in experiments on animals. What people drink is not pure alcohol, and possibly alcohol produces its carcinogenic effects only when accompanied by other substances.

Various studies have shown correlations between alcoholic drinks and cancers of the oesophagus, larynx, liver and mouth; the alcohol perhaps not acting as a direct carcinogen but helping to transport carcinogens in the bloodstream.

Alcohol and tobacco, as well as independently increasing the risk of some cancers, appear also to combine to increase each other's harmful influence. Tobacco certainly represents the greater danger, however, and for people who do not smoke there is very little, if any, cancer risk from alcohol.

diet

There is now no doubt that we risk cancer when we draw tobacco smoke into our lungs, and it may be supposed that cancer of the digestive organs is similarly connected with the food we put into them. The evidence that this is so is, however, weak and very little can be said with confidence. It is possible to show that some populations eating large amounts of some foods have a certain cancer pattern. There are some reasons for thinking that these may contribute to the production of the disease, but the evidence is far from conclusive. It is hard to establish exactly what, and how much, people have been eating; and most cancers suspected of being related to diet develop over a long period of time, so that it is not easy to match cause and effect.

It is known that cancers can be induced in experimental animals by altering their diets in various ways. Such laboratory evidence is helpful but it has not yet clearly pointed to any specific elements of the human diet – other than to a harmful effect of overeating.

It is therefore very difficult to determine exactly how diet can induce cancer in man. Several mechanisms – not mutually exclusive – have been suggested.

food which causes cancer?

There is a limited amount of evidence pointing to this or that food as containing an identifiable carcinogen – but none of these foods is important in Britain. Bracken fern is commonly eaten in parts of Japan that also have a high incidence of oesophageal cancer and has been linked to the development of the disease. Cows which feed on this fern are found to develop gastric cancers, and their milk has induced cancer in laboratory rats. It is most probable, then, that some component of the fern is a carcinogen: but opinion is divided about which one it is and how it acts. It has not been linked to any cancer in Britain. Rotted salted fish that is commonly eaten in southern China almost certainly helps to cause the cancer of the nose that occurs there.

Nitrous compounds, such as sodium or potassium nitrate or nitrite, are used in smoking and curing meat, for instance, ham, bacon, salt beef, and have been suspected of causing cancer. They are probably harmless in themselves, but it is possible that they are converted by the body into nitrosamines, shown by laboratory evidence to be carcinogenic. They have not, however, been clearly linked to the development of any cancers in humans.

In Britain, the principal sources of nitrates are fresh vegetables, but these generally seem to be protective against cancer, possibly because the creation of nitrosamines is inhibited by the presence of ascorbic acid (vitamin C) and alpha-tocopherol (vitamin E) and possibly for other reasons.

cooking methods?

Suspicion has fallen on polycyclic aromatic hydrocarbons, compounds arising from a number of sources, such as incomplete combustion of organic substances and the resulting pollution. They are found in just about every sort of food but are particularly produced in foods that have been smoked, or cooked at high temperatures, such as grilled or roasted. Some of these compounds have been found to cause cancer in laboratory animals. However, there is no definite epidemiological evidence linking any human cancers to the eating of smoked meat and fish and to the grilled and barbecued meats that are eaten in huge quantities throughout the United States, where the incidence of stomach cancer is actually falling faster than in Britain.

storage

In some cases, a cancer hazard results from the storage of foodstuffs. Moulds often grow in storage: some moulds produce toxic compounds called mycotoxins. At least one of these, aflatoxin, is an important contributing cause of cancer of the liver. The moulds that produce aflatoxin can grow on oil-rich foods, particularly on peanuts and maize, and people for whom these are a staple food are particularly at risk. This is the case in Africa and parts of China and Thailand, where there is a strong association between aflatoxin in foods and very high rates of liver cancer.

fats in the food

Studies of the incidence of cancer in different countries have demonstrated a close correlation between the proportion of fat in the diet and the incidence of cancer of the breast in women, cancer of the prostate in men, and of the large bowel (colon and rectum) in both. There is partial confirmation of this in a study of Japanese women migrants to the United States. The proportion of fat in the traditional Japanese diet is low, and so is the incidence of breast cancer; this stays much the same in first-generation migrants (which may show the importance of early eating habits). In the following generation, brought up on the American high-fat style of eating, breast cancer rates in Japanese women reach the high all-American levels. What is more, breast cancer in Japan itself is on the increase, as more of the native population comes to adopt the American way of eating.

Japanese migrants to Hawaii similarly show higher rates of prostate and bowel cancer than Japanese in Japan.

The link between dietary fat and cancer has been supported by some experimental work on animals. But studies designed to find out whether, within a given country, people who develop cancers have eaten more fat than people who are cancer-free, have given inconclusive results.

It is not certain, from animal experiments, whether fat itself has any specific effect or whether such effects as there are, derive from the fact that fat is such a high source of calories.

Fat may, in fact, be implicated in both ways. In the case of the bowel, fat consumption increases the secretion of bile steroids and bile acids (secreted by the liver to aid the digestion of fat) and chemicals derived from these secretions may possibly act to promote cancer. In the case of the breast and prostate, both of which are glands regulated by hormones, a cancer risk could result from hormones secreted by body fat.

It is not known whether the kind of fat that is eaten – animal or vegetable, saturated or polyunsaturated – makes any difference.

how much you eat

Animals, like human beings, are more likely to develop cancer as they grow older. However, it has been known for many years that laboratory animals fed on a sparse diet are less likely to develop tumours, and so live longer than those that are allowed to eat their fill. Consequently, a link has been suggested between calorie intake and cancer, but it is not established whether the important factor is the total calorie level, or the fat level (which tends to be low in a low-calorie diet), or some other factor.

In human beings, the evidence is indirect and not wholly conclusive. It is based on studies of the effect of obesity on cancer rates. The best documented examples are those of cancer of the gall bladder and endometrium (lining of the womb). The endometrium is hormone-dependent: that is, it is influenced by the body's levels of oestrogen (the female sex hormone). The tumour tends to occur in obese women after the menopause, when normally the secretion of oestrogen should dwindle, but it is possible that the fat tissues then become important sources of oestrogen. Endometrial cancer is similarly known to develop in post-menopausal women who are receiving oestrogen therapy.

Another potential effect of a diet high in calories is that of inducing early menarche (start of puberty and menstruation). The well-fed girls of western society start to menstruate earlier in life than their third-world counterparts; they also tend to start childbearing much later. There is evidence of an association between an increased rate of breast cancer and this long gap between menarche and first baby.

food additives

As people have been becoming more aware of the actual constitutents of what they eat, and as 'natural' foods have come to be particularly esteemed, food additives have come under suspicion of causing cancer and other diseases.

Hundreds of substances with alarmingly chemical names are added as preservatives or 'improvers' to a great variety of foods. Any new additive (such as new sweeteners) must undergo stringent tests for causing cancer, but some customary additives (including 'natural' ones) have never been put to the test. The following, however, have been tested – but with no conclusive results.

saccharin
is the only current artificial additive known to be able to cause cancer experimentally. It has been found to induce bladder cancer in male rats when administered in huge doses which no human intake could equal. It continues to be used because many studies have failed to demonstrate that it has any harmful effect in humans.

butylated hydroxytoluene
is a food additive, an antioxidant with preservative properties. This is not a carcinogen: it may even help to prevent stomach cancer.

PVC (polyvinyl chloride)
Nobody actually adds this to food, but it has been found that minute amounts of the vinyl chloride of which it is composed leach out from PVC containers into the food inside. Workers in vinyl chloride manufacture who used to be heavily exposed, underwent a risk of a cancer of the liver. But there is no evidence that the tiny amounts that find their way into food have caused cancer in domestic users of PVC containers.

plastic food wrap
Recently, doubt has been cast on clear plastic food-wrapping film. Additives called plasticisers, used in its manufacture, leach out into food wrapped in it, and some American laboratory trials have suggested a link between them and cancer in mice. Not enough research has yet been done in this field to know whether human beings would be affected.

This is mostly true also of the whole field of food additives; the case against them is not proven.

how great is the risk?
It has been estimated that in the USA anything between 10 and 70 per cent of all cancer deaths may be related to diet in one way or another, and the same is true of Britain. The wide range of estimates show how much there is still to be learned about this subject.

sex-life and childbearing

Where these two related activities are concerned, participation and abstention both seem to carry their own cancer risks.

For women, there is a premium in chastity: cancer of the cervix (neck of the womb) is very rare in life-long virgins, such as nuns. The risk is highest for women who have many partners: prostitutes, for instance, and those who begin to have sex early in life, presumably because they are likely to have many partners.

This strongly suggests that cervical cancer results from something passed on to the woman by the man. The carcinogenic agent may be a virus present in semen. Some other factor may be involved, such as papilloma viruses which cause genital warts, and there is also an association with the herpes virus. Studies have suggested that the risk of cancer is high not only for promiscuous women (who have multiple chances of exposure) but also for women who have only one partner if he is himself promiscuous.

It is not fully explained why the wives of Jewish husbands have a low incidence of cervical cancer; it has been thought to be because their husbands are circumcised, but circumcision does not seem to protect against this disease in many other cultures. Some people believe that it was because Jewish husbands and wives have tended not to have extramarital partners. Now that is no longer the case, the incidence is rising.

A cause-and-effect relationship has been suggested between cervical cancer and the contraceptive pill. The age at which a woman starts taking the pill may be a factor. There is now evidence that taking the pill for more than 5 or even 3 years increases the risk of cervical cancer to a small extent (though the association may be due to more extensive sexual activity of women taking the pill). Also whether the woman smokes may be a factor.

It is generally agreed, however, that taking the pill reduces the risk of cancer of the womb and of the ovaries. Ovarian cancer is also less frequent in women who have had children. It is possible that the suppression of ovulation during pregnancy reduces the chances of malignancy, and more pregnancies enhance protection. The contraceptive pill, which also suppresses ovulation, may act in the same way.

There is an increased risk of breast cancer for women who have not borne children by the age of 30. Full-term pregnancy seems to offer a degree of protection, if it occurs early in life. At a later age (after 35 or so) it may increase the risk.

occupational risks

Some trades and manufactures are known to entail a significant risk of cancer to the people who work in them. The earliest documented instance is the observation by the surgeon Percival Pott, in 1775, that chimney-sweeps' climbing-boys, who had soot rubbed into every part of their bodies (they worked naked), had a high chance of developing cancer of the scrotum.

Since then, many types of cancer have been associated with various occupations. One of the best attested is that mesothelioma, that is, cancer of the membrane which lines the chest and abdominal cavity, is caused by exposure to asbestos. Other examples are: leukaemia caused by benzene in rubber manufacture (amongst others); bladder cancer caused by some of the chemicals used in the dye industry and, to a lesser degree, by benzidine (now banned in Britain); scrotal cancer caused by cutting oils used by metal workers. Ionising radiation, known to cause all types of cancer, is an occupational risk for some workers in the health services and the nuclear industry. Nasal cancer is commonest where hardwood furniture is made: it is associated with wood dust.

There has been much argument about what proportion of cancers in the United Kingdom are occupational in origin: it now seems unlikely to be more than 1 in 25 (that is 4% of all cancers). Precise estimates are difficult to make because there is also the effect of smoking and many industrial workers smoke.

sunlight

Excessive exposure to sunlight is an important cause of several types of skin cancer: basal cell carcinoma (rodent ulcer), a slow-growing non-invasive cancer on the face and neck; squamous carcinoma in any of the cells of the skin; and, most dangerous of all, malignant melanoma, which arises from the cells which produce brown pigment. The cancer-causing agent is the ultra violet (UV) radiation in sunlight, which damages the DNA of skin cells. Very fair-skinned people are most at risk, especially if they do outdoor work, such as farming.

Melanoma is greatly on the increase among light-skinned people in many parts of the world, due, probably, to the admiration and prestige that go with a deep suntan.

pollution

This is a general term for the contamination – mostly man-made – of the three props of life on earth: air, water and food. Many of the contaminants are potentially carcinogenic. Estimates of the extent of pollution and of the damage it does are complicated because there are so many contaminants, several of which are likely to be at work in any one instance; because the amounts to which people are exposed are generally very small; and because the effects are likely to become apparent only after a long time.

atmospheric pollution
The air we breathe is contaminated by countless foreign substances. Amongst them are polycyclic aromatic hydrocarbons (products of incomplete combustion, already mentioned in connection with diet): we inhale the variety called benzpyrenes in the form of soot and tar from the combustion of coal and oil. We also inhale asbestos fibres, lead from car exhausts, chemicals from industrial processes, tobacco tars from other people's smoking ('passive smoking'), and much else. However, it is not clear how much all this contributes to the cancer statistics.

It has been thought that air pollution contributed to lung cancer, because the mortality rate for cigarette-smoking town dwellers has been twice that of smokers in the country. However, non-smokers in town have the same low incidence of lung cancer as those in the country. The explanation of this is probably that present-day lung cancer rates reflect the smoking habits of 40 or more years ago, when smoking was much less common in the country than in the more 'sophisticated' towns.

Fluorocarbons, the propellant gases in aerosol sprays, have been investigated because of a suspicion that their combined effect could be destroying some of the ozone layer surrounding the earth, so letting more UV radiation through, with a consequent increase in skin cancers. This hypothesis has never been proved and some evidence now suggests that it is unlikely to be true.

water pollution
The sophisticated techniques now available to analytical chemists are able to reveal the presence of contaminants in our drinking water even when these occur in minute concentrations: they include pesticides, asbestos fibres (from asbestos cement pipes), vinyl chloride (from PVC pipes), arsenic and radioactive compounds (both naturally occurring and from industrial sources). Though these are all potential carcinogens, none has been found in concentrations sufficient in themselves to offer a danger to health. However, it is not known whether there are any safe levels of exposure to any carcinogen, and if several of these contaminants are present, their combined effect may be greater

than the sum of the individual effects. Up to now there is no evidence to show that drinking water makes any contribution to cancer incidence even though water is also 'contaminated' by chlorination, to purify it.

As far as fluoridation (to reduce the incidence of tooth decay) is concerned, where it has been possible to monitor the effects of this in this country, in areas with static populations, there has been no observable effect on cancer incidence.

food pollution

Pollutants of food include sewage and industrial effluent in sea water, which contaminate fish; pesticides in fruit and vegetables; and polycyclic hydrocarbons in almost everything. Though these may be potential carcinogens, experimental confirmation is hard to obtain without feeding these substances to laboratory animals in amounts far greater than a human being would ingest in his normal diet. As in the case of water, it is hard to estimate what the effects of a lifetime's consumption would be, but there is no evidence that they add significantly to cancer incidence.

radiation

That ionising radiation resulting from nuclear fission induces cancer is attested by the experience of survivors of Hiroshima and Nagasaki. The danger of prolonged exposure to X-rays is also well documented, and it is generally agreed that the use of diagnostic X-rays should be kept to an essential minimum.

Ionising radiation is an occupational risk for workers in hospital radiology departments and in nuclear power stations (such as Sizewell) and plants reprocessing nuclear waste (such as Sellafield, formerly Windscale) and even more so in the older type Magnox reactors.

Some ionising radiation also occurs naturally as cosmic rays and is given off everywhere by the earth and all buildings.

A study carried out by the Atomic Energy Authority among its workers has shown an overall incidence of cancer well within the expected range and lower than the national average – probably because the workers are generally healthier than the average population. It does not mean that work in a nuclear energy establishment has beneficial effects and reduces cancer incidence. The reason for the reduced incidence among workers compared with the national average is because the latter includes chronically ill people who would not be accepted for a job in the industry. This is known as a 'selection' factor. There was, however, a possibly higher than expected incidence of some individual types of cancer, such as leukaemia, cancer of the prostate, and cancer of the testicles.

Workers in the nuclear industry have protective clothing and shielding, and their exposure to radiation is monitored. However, this is not the case for members of the public who live near nuclear installations and are at risk from accidental discharges of radioactive materials, as at Windscale in 1957 and Sellafield recently. A small excess of childhood leukaemia has now been reported in the vicinity of at least three major nuclear plants.

Conclusive evidence is lacking and will probably be hard to obtain.

In conclusion, even if all sources of pollution (with the exception of smoking) are aggregated, their combined effect could be held responsible for a very small percentage of all cancer mortality.

The effects of the disaster at Chernobyl, in the USSR, in April 1986, are not yet known.

infection and immunity

An interest in the possible role of viruses (disease-causing micro-organisms) as the cause of cancer is being revived by the discovery of the important role that the hepatitis B virus plays in causing cancer of the liver. Carriers of the viral particles may be free of hepatitis symptoms but are at significant risk (100 times that of non-carriers) of developing hepatoma (liver cancer), usually in their twenties or thirties. This cancer is a major health problem in the third-world countries where hepatitis is endemic.

There is also the association of the E-B (Epstein-Barr) virus with Burkitt's lymphoma (a cancer of the lymph glands which is common in parts of Africa and China).

Also, there is the identification of a lymphoid cancer occurring in unusual groups of cases in the same area, in parts of Japan and the Caribbean. A virus has been discovered (HTLV-I) that is probably responsible for the transformation of the normal lymphoid cells into cancer cells.

Although viruses have long been known to cause cancers in animals, it has only recently been accepted that these three viruses (E-B, hepatitis B and HTLV-I) are important for human cancers and it is possible that several other cancers also stem from a virus infection. There must be other contributory factors as well, because many people are infected by these viruses, yet relatively few contract cancer. Possibly some people will have an immune response to the virus; or some other factors may intervene.

There is also the discovery that some types of the human papilloma virus can nearly always be found in cancer of the cervix: there is now much evidence to suggest that this is also a virus-induced cancer.

The now notorious AIDS (acquired immune deficiency syndrome) is the result of a virus infection (HTLV-III). It causes a collapse of part of the body's immune system (which fights infection), and sometimes leads to a hitherto rare and aggressive cancer, Kaposi's sarcoma.

For many years it has been suspected that lowered immunity can predispose to certain cancers. Evidence of this is the incidence of some particular cancers in people who have received transplants of kidneys and other organs. In them, the immune system is deliberately depressed by drugs, to keep the body from identifying as 'non-self' the donated organs and rejecting them. Consequently, it may also fail to identify and destroy a cancer-causing virus.

modern medicine

Paradoxically, exposure to certain anti-cancer drugs may ulti-
mately increase the risk of a second cancer. Malignant diseases
have occasionally, but according to a predictable pattern, been
shown to occur several years after exposure to the anti-cancer
drugs which cured the original disease.

Diagnostic X-rays probably do not do much harm to the vast
majority of patients; the amount of exposure received in the
course of an average investigation is not likely to be harmful, but
since the effect of exposure is cumulative, an excessive number
of X-rays should be avoided. (There is, for example, an association of the start of breast cancer and multiple diagnostic X-rays).

THE PREVENTION OF CANCER

This is a difficult topic, for several reasons. First, we still have no clear idea of exactly how a normal cell is turned into a cancer cell; in many cases the mechanism of causation remains a mystery. Neither do we know exactly what particular ways of living are associated with some kinds of cancer. There is always the possibility of the erroneous supposition that because two events occur in succession, the second was caused by the first. It may be that both of them are the result of some other cause. Some of the associations that have been observed may turn out to be secondary: for instance, the association between obesity and cancer of the breast may turn out to be coincidental, and some other factor may be responsible for both.

Statistics based on epidemiological studies strongly suggest that doing or not doing certain things may reduce or increase one's chances of contracting cancer. It is, however, difficult to prove that something has been prevented by something else, that is, to prove a negative.

Though there may be good evidence pointing to some of the practices of our daily lives as causing cancer, it is not enough simply to tell people to abstain from them. One can rightly urge people to stop smoking and to drink moderately, but it is impracticable to tell them to stop breathing polluted city air and other people's cigarette smoke, or to throw up their jobs in machine shops and foundries. Nor are parents in Europe likely to press their daughters to marry and have children as soon after menarche as the law allows, simply in the hope of saving them from breast cancer in the future.

giving up smoking

A good many smokers do not get lung cancer, and what is more, a few non-smokers do. Similarly, some careless drivers live to a ripe old age, and some careful ones die in road accidents, but this does not make careless driving a sensible policy. The vast majority of lung cancer victims have been heavy smokers. So, a wise person will not smoke. All the evidence suggests that total abstention is the best policy. Switching to low-tar cigarettes reduces the risk of lung cancer but it may or may not reduce the risk of other cancers (for example, of the mouth and bladder) and other smoking-related diseases. Switching to pipes and cigars is likely to be of even less help, partly (but not solely) because it is difficult to alter habits of inhaling.

cutting down on alcohol
It seems that in the absence of smoking, a moderate alcohol consumption is unlikely to increase the risk of cancer. Greater consumption is inadvisable for many other reasons also.

diet

The association between a diet rich in fat and some types of cancer suggests that it may be helpful to reduce severely one's overall consumption of fat. This is almost bound to lower one's total calorie intake, since fats supply, ounce for ounce, more than twice as many calories as proteins or carbohydrates and it does seem that keeping to a moderate intake of calories is a clue to a healthy and extended life. Even if it does not reduce greatly the risk of cancer, it will probably reduce the risk of heart disease. Some people think it wise to eat as little as possible of smoked, cured, salted and pickled foods, as this may reduce one's chances of cancer of the stomach. Others, however, think it would have little if any effect.

This is the 'don't' side of dietary prevention: there are some things one should probably 'do' – eat more of, or, at least, not exclude from one's diet altogether.

dietary fibre

This is a general name for the substances such as cellulose, lignin, pectin, gums and pentose polymers which act as the supporting structure or 'skeleton' of wholegrain cereals, fruit and vegetables. They are not digested by the human digestive system, and so add very few calories to the diet, only bulk. Wheat bran is probably the best known source of fibre, because it is widely sold in the form of breakfast cereals, but vegetable fibre is also important.

Fibre was formerly known as 'roughage'; preoccupation with it used to be associated with food cranks. The pioneering work of Dr Denis Burkitt, and subsequent studies, have, however, demonstrated that many populations in the 'developing' countries, whose diet contains a great deal of fibre, have a low incidence of cancer of the colon, compared with people in the western countries, who eat foods from which the fibre has mostly been refined: white flour and polished rice, for instance.

How fibre helps is not known exactly. There are several theories. One is that fibre reduces intestinal 'transit time', that is, it increases the rate at which food waste passes through the bowel, and so any carcinogenic substances in the waste do not remain long in contact with the colon wall. Another theory suggests that the added bulk from the fibre, plus the water which it readily absorbs, serve to dilute the harmful substances. Yet another theory is that the presence of fibre increases the quantity of colonic flora (micro-organisms which break down food residue) and makes them cope better with carcinogens.

However, epidemiological evidence has thrown some doubt on the dietary fibre theory. It is now suggested that fibre is protective if you eat a high fat diet, but less important if you eat a low fat diet.

Whatever the case, there is little doubt that it is a good idea to include plenty of fibre in one's diet. No need to add bran to everything: it is more sensible to choose wholegrain bread and brown rice in preference to the white kinds, and to eat plenty of pulses (beans, lentils, etc.), vegetables and fruit.

Such a diet is nowadays also widely recommended to help prevent and control some other scourges of the western world – obesity, maturity-onset diabetes and coronary heart disease – so there is everything to be said for it.

vitamin A

This occurs in its pure form, as retinol, in some foods of animal origin: for example, liver, whole milk and butter (by law, it is added to margarine). It is found in carrots and in dark green and yellow vegetables and also some fruit, such as apricots and persimmons, in the form of beta-carotene and other carotinoids which are converted in the body into retinol.

Great interest was aroused by numerous epidemiological studies which showed a relationship between high beta-carotene consumption and a reduced incidence of lung cancer in men, and also of cancers of the bladder, oesophagus and stomach. These, like the majority of cancers, originate in the epithelium, the tissue of which the skin and the lining of internal organs are composed. A deficiency of vitamin A causes a reduction of differentiation in the epithelial cells, similar to that which occurs in cancer cells. It was thought that a high level of vitamin A in the blood (serum retinol) might help to prevent contact with carcinogens from bringing about such loss of differentiation. In some animal experiments, retinol has even been shown to arrest, to some extent, damage done to cells by chemical carcinogens.

Recent research has, however, contradicted some of the early findings and it is now clear that in Britain and the usa the level of retinol in the blood has no effect on the incidence of any cancer. It is still possible, however, that beta-carotene may produce some benefit.

The eating of green and yellow vegetables and fruit may do good in several other ways, partly because they provide a source of vitamin C and partly because of other components which have not yet been identified in detail. More will be known about the possible beneficial effects of these substances when the trials are finished that are now being carried out in the usa, using men doctors as subjects, to test the effects of beta-carotene (and other subjects to test the effect of vitamin C and other substances).

Taken in excess (which it is possible to do by drinking very large quantities of carrot juice, for example), beta-carotene can turn the skin yellow and have other unpleasant effects. It is harmless when taken in the form of large amounts of yellow or green fruit and vegetables. However, retinol itself is definitely toxic in excess amounts. (It is, for example, very unwise to dose oneself freely with vitamin A pills.)

vitamin C (ascorbic acid)

Important claims have been made for this vitamin; that it not only has a part to play in preventing cancer, but is able, in huge doses, to slow down and even arrest the progress of tumours already formed.

There is some epidemiological backing for the first claim: the high incidence of cancers of the stomach in some populations has been associated with a low vitamin C intake – in Iceland, for example, and some parts of Great Britain. But it is hard to be sure how this protection comes about, because the evidence depends on the consumption of fruit and vegetables, which also supply beta-carotene, fibre and other potentially beneficial components.

Vitamin C is an anti-oxidant, able to prevent the conversion of nitrates and nitrites into carcinogenic nitrosamines, and it seems possible that eating plenty of foods rich in vitamin C – such as citrus fruits – may protect against cancer of the stomach and oesophagus.

As for the vitamin's alleged power to arrest the spread of cancer, trials have been carried out in the USA, in which some cancer patients were given doses of ascorbic acid, and others doses of a placebo (dummy) preparation, and their survival rates compared. The results of these trials have been claimed to demolish the case for vitamin C, but they have been criticised on methodological grounds, and the question is by no means settled. Until more is known, it is probably prudent to take vitamin C in the form of fruit and vegetables, thus also getting the benefits of fibre and beta-carotene, rather than in the enormous doses of ascorbic acid in tablet form recommended by some of its advocates. For a woman on the pill it is not desirable to take large doses of vitamin C because some research has suggested that this converts a low-oestrogen pill to a high dose pill.

vitamin E (alpha-tocopherol)

This, too, has anti-oxidant properties, and is able to inhibit the formation of nitrosamines and could thus be important in preventing cancer. It is the fat-soluble counterpart of vitamin C (which is water-soluble) and so is found in many foods with a fat content, such as vegetable oils, wheatgerm and other foods based on whole grains, also eggs, nuts and some vegetables. It has therefore been supposed that it is difficult for people to have a deficiency of it. But it tends to deteriorate in storage, and is sometimes destroyed by processing – as when the oils are refined – so that it is not easy to know how much one is getting.

A modest daily supplement of vitamin E (in capsule form) may be a good idea, especially when one's diet includes a good proportion of polyunsaturated fats in the form of refined vegetable oils. But it has no curative effect and additional vitamin E should be avoided where a hormone-dependent cancer (such as of testicles, breast, ovary) has already been diagnosed.

selenium

This is a trace element present in many foods, such as whole grains, milk, eggs and some vegetables, including onions and tomatoes. It is derived from the soil in which crops are grown. People in areas in which selenium levels in the soil are low are likely to have a low selenium level in the blood. There is some evidence that low levels of selenium in the blood are associated with a higher risk of cancer, but it is very weak. The subject is now being studied and within a few years it should be known whether or not it is of any importance.

In any event, because selenium is present in so many foods, it should be unnecessary to take supplementary doses. But there is no way of knowing exactly how much selenium there is in one's food. Anyone thinking of taking a supplement should make sure it does not exceed 200 micrograms a day. Selenium is toxic in high doses.

In conclusion, all that can safely be said about the role of food in the prevention of cancer, boils down to this: the best kind of daily diet is low in fat of all kinds, and includes plenty of wholegrain bread and cereals, fruit and vegetables. This is a regime which most nutritionists would recommend on several different counts.

contraception

Because of the continuing suspicion that the contraceptive pill may promote cervical cancer, it may be prudent to consider changing to a 'barrier' method of contraception: the sheath or the diaphragm (particularly if a woman over 35 has been taking the pill for a long time). Women on the contraceptive pill should make sure that they have regular cervical smear tests. Whatever one may consider to be their drawbacks, the sheath and diaphragm present no danger to health, in the short or long term; indeed, they may even offer some small protection against the transfer of a virus or some other cancer-forming agent from one partner to the other. They are, however, less convenient and less effective forms of contraception and individual people are likely to judge the balance of risk and benefit differently.

occupational risks

As mentioned before, some industrial processes involve a cancer risk for the workers. The advice to get another kind of work is not generally practicable: but there are ways of minimising the risks in the work one has got. In most trades, there are protective measures such as shielding, special clothing, health checks, which are prescribed by law and enforced by inspectors. It is up to the workers to insist, through the medium of their trade union or otherwise, on the rigid application of all precautions and monitoring, and on getting all the protection that is due to them and applying the safety precautions themselves.

sunbathing

Fair-skinned people with blond or red hair and blue eyes usually have low levels of melanin, the brown pigmentation which appears in response to sunlight to protect the skin. They would be wise to keep out of bright sunlight, or, if they must sunbathe, to choose times when the sun is not at its fiercest (at midday, for example), and to use a sunscreen with a protection factor of 10 or more, able to screen out UV rays. Using a sunscreen which merely prevents burning may not be enough.

conclusion

If it is difficult to establish what causes many of the cancers, it is even more difficult to discover what does not. There is no human activity that carries a guarantee of complete safety, or that can be positively stated to confer immunity: in fact, since the development of tumours is associated with ageing, it could be said that being alive is an occupation with a cancer risk. All that any of us can do is to consider the balance of probabilities, in so far as it can be known, and make life choices on this basis. Remember that avoiding smoking will do more good than all the other suggested methods of preventing cancer combined.

THE PROBLEM OF DETECTING EARLY CANCER

In its earliest stages, a cancer usually has no symptoms. By the time it is giving rise to unmistakable warning signals, it will usually have grown large enough to be visible to the doctor, either with the naked eye, or with the help of X-rays or of an endoscope (an instrument for looking inside the stomach, the intestine and other hollow organs).

This means that the cancer will now probably be a lump one-half to one centimetre in diameter; say, as big as a hazelnut (though it could be very much larger). It will comprise anything between a hundred million and a thousand million cells, representing 30 generations from the original cancer cell. After a further thirteen generations (between a million million and ten million million cells) the cancer will have become something like a kilogram in weight or a litre in volume, at which stage it would usually be fatal. (Not all cancers manifest themselves as lumps – for instance, leukaemias and mesotheliomas do not. Some stomach cancers are sheets of cells, not lumps, but the principle of cell multiplication is much the same.)

Purely in terms of cell multiplication, then, if a cancer is not detected until it is causing unmistakable symptoms this can be likened to recognising the existence of a new individual, not at gestation, nor even at birth, but somewhere in early middle age. The significance of this invisible infancy, youth and young adulthood of a cancer has implications for the individual that vary with the cancer. Some cancers develop rapidly, so that the time span from inception to fatal termination can be measured in weeks. Others grow much more slowly, and may take years to develop from the initial malignant cell to the detectable cancer.

screening for cancer – the pros and cons

It has been repeatedly demonstrated that the earlier the disease is diagnosed, the easier it is to treat and the greater is the likelihood of controlling and possibly even curing it. Because of the potential value of early detection, much deliberation has gone into deciding how useful and effective programmes of screening are.

Obviously, screening could only be for the commonest types of cancer: it would be impracticable to screen everyone for everything. An analogy can be made with screening for pulmonary tuberculosis. Screening costs money, but thirty years ago, making chest X-rays available to the whole population was considered worthwhile, for two reasons: tuberculosis was a common ailment, and a cure had been found for it, provided it was detected early. Consequently, the benefit of screening was enormous, and fully justified the cost of mass X-ray units. As the incidence of TB began to decline, for various reasons, it was no longer worthwhile to X-ray everyone, and screening was offered only to people at high risk of contracting the disease.

Lung cancer might be thought to be an obvious candidate for screening because the cancer is common; the detection technique (basically chest X-rays) is still relatively cheap and widely available, and there is a well-defined high-risk group (i.e. cigarette smokers).

Unfortunately screening has been shown not to pick up a sufficient number of lung tumours early enough to make it worthwhile, and repeated X-rays of the chest would cause more cancers than they would get cured. Lung cancer is by no means as curable as tuberculosis became after the discovery of antibiotics.

And when it comes to the generality of cancers, the question is also not so straightforward, for the following reasons:

○ There is no single test that could be routinely used to screen for all types of cancer.

○ Tests that can disprove or prove the presence of a cancer are not simple or inexpensive.
○ No cancer is as widespread as tuberculosis was when screening for it was introduced.

Thus, the usefulness of screening is very different indeed for such very different types of cancer. With the fast-growing sort, it is most unlikely that the screening of any given patient would pick up the disease during the brief interval between becoming detectable and becoming untreatable. The occasional, random success would not make the test worthwhile.

Some kinds of cancer are so rare that mass screening could never be economically justified. Others are hard to detect because their site of origin is not easily accessible to screening. Any of these arguments may, singly or together, be applied to many cancers.

However, there are several cancers which appear to be suitable candidates for screening, because they are common; are associated with defined high-risk groups; can be detected by means of an appropriate screening technique or because there is a pre-cancerous condition which can be recognised and treated.

The question to ask then is: should these techniques be made available to all members of the high-risk groups? The answer must be to a large extent financial: screening costs money, and the financing from public sources will not be forthcoming unless it can be shown that wide-scale screening will mean, not only many more cancers detected, but also many more cancers successfully treated.

Where the prospects of successful treatment are poor, widespread screening at the public expense is unlikely to be thought worthwhile. This argument will seem unfair to those who are denied screening unless they pay for it themselves.

cervical cancer

There is one type of cancer for which the rewards of screening can be enormous. This is cancer of the neck of the womb (cervix uteri), and is virtually confined to women who are or have been sexually active. It may appear as early as 20 years but is commonest in women over thirty-five. It is nearly always preceded by the appearance of abnormal, 'pre-malignant' cells, and may take ten or more years to progress to the dangerous, invasive stage. Consequently a delay in detecting it may not be absolutely critical.

The abnormal cells can be destroyed easily by one of several techniques which offer the sufferer an excellent chance of complete recovery, with no reduction of her chances of bearing children.

The smear test (often called the Pap test, after Dr George Papanicolaou, its inventor) is simple and should be painless. A vaginal examination is followed by a gentle scraping of the cervix with a wooden spatula; the doctor (or nurse) then transfers the scraped cells on to a slide, and sends them to a cytological laboratory (one equipped to scrutinise cells). The laboratory examination is quite quick to do: new techniques are being developed to make it yet faster and more foolproof.

Health authorities or health boards are recommended by the DHSS to make the smear test available every three to five years to women in the high-risk age group (from 35 years). Many young women are also tested as a matter of routine when pregnant, or in family planning clinics or when seeing the GP for a pill prescription. University health services generally make cervical screening available to their women students.

However, the incidence of cervical cancer in women under thirty-five is on the increase (from 15 per cent of all cervical cancer cases in 1972, to 27 per cent in 1982), and in some of them it has seemed to take a more aggressive form. The malignant cells are of the anaplastic, rapidly growing kind, and are markedly invasive, so that, unless observed early, the disease is likely to develop beyond control.

This is one reason for the depressing nature of the cervical cancer statistics, which show that more than 2,000 women a year still die of this disease. Amongst the other important reasons is that the health service laboratories are in many areas unable to cope with the demand for their services, and have a backlog of smears waiting to be examined, with a consequent delay between test and treatment which, in the case of the aggressive form of cervical cancer, may prove critical.

A debate is going on about the best way of allocating the scarce screening resources. One side of the argument contends that free smear tests should be made available to younger women also – idealy, twice at a year's interval and then every three years – because for them time is of the essence. Another school of thought insists that cervical cancer in young women is still comparatively rare, and that available resources should be concentrated on more frequent and efficient testing for the older women. Another point of view is that the screening services are being overwhelmed by repeat smears of women who are less at risk than others (mainly social class I and II).

While this question is being thrashed out, the wisest course for any woman who has not had a smear test for more than two or three years (or never had one at all) is to insist on having one as soon as practicable. This is especially advisable for women who have reached the years of danger and for someone who (or whose partner) has had genital herpes or genital warts (which predispose to cancer of the cervix), and long-term users of the pill. Going to one's own doctor should be a starting point. If there is no help to be had there, other possibilities are: self-referral to local authority welfare clinics; family planning clinics; well-woman clinics. Information about these is usually available at the public library, or at the town hall and citizens advice bureaux.

INSPECTION - How to look

Undressed to the waist, sit in front of a mirror
in a good light.

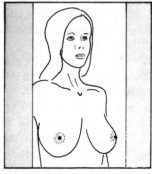

1 LOOK: hands at your sides
or on your hips, look carefully
at your breasts. Turn from
side to side. Look underneath
too.

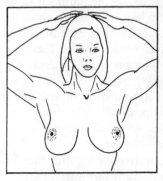

2 LIFT: hands on your head,
look for anything unusual,
especially around the nipple.

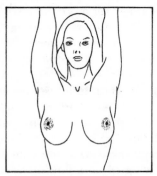

3 STRETCH: arms stretched
above your head, look again,
particularly around the nipple.

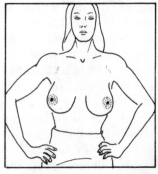

4 PRESS: hands on hips, press
inwards until your chest muscles
tighten. Look again, especially
for any dimpling of the skin.

Task 1

breast cancer

In Britain, breast cancer is the commonest cancer in women. It occurs in about one woman in seventeen, and is the cause of some 12,000 deaths a year.

Most types of breast cancer metastasise readily, so the likelihood that treatment will be successful in bringing about a cure is greatest for patients in whom the disease is detected early. About 30 per cent of women in whom cancer is detected early will, after treatment, have a normal life expectation. Overall, for women with breast cancer the average survival rate is about 10 years.

The early disease (before it has spread) is straightforward to treat. The more advanced the disease is, the more drastic are the measures required and the lower are the chances of success.

There are three methods of detection in current use. The first is self-examination: this is recommended as a routine monthly procedure (immediately after each period) for all women and specially recommended to the highest-risk group, women who are approaching or have passed through the menopause and those whose mother or sisters have had breast cancer.

The breasts are inspected in a mirror for any visible changes, such as dimpling, puckering, nipple retraction, or any changes in size or shape; they are then palpated, that is, felt all over with the flat of the fingers, in order to detect any lumps.

Detailed instruction in the technique can be had from one's medical practitioner, from local well-woman clinics, family planning clinics and from self-help organisations. The Womens National Cancer Control Campaign (1 South Audley Street, London WIY 5DQ) has a free illustrated leaflet (on which these illustrations are based) with detailed instructions on how to do self-examination properly.

This 'screening' method has the advantage of costing nothing and being available to all – even though very small lumps may be missed.

PALPATION - How to feel

Lie on a flat surface, head on a pillow, shoulder slightly raised by a folded towel.

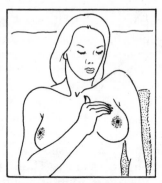

1 Left shoulder raised, feel the left breast with the right hand. Use the flat of the fingers, keeping them together.

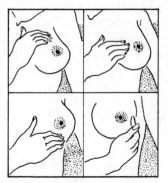

2 Press the breast gently but firmly in towards the body. Work in a spiral, circling out from the nipple. Feel every part.

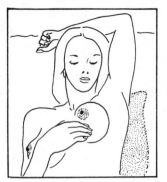

3 Left arm above your head, elbow bent, repeat the spiral carefully. Feel the outer part of the breast especially.

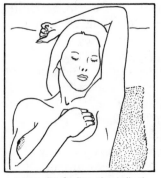

4 Finish by feeling the tail of the breast towards the armpit. Repeat all four stages on the other breast. Be thorough. Don't rush.

The second method is examination by a doctor or nurse, which, as well as visual inspection and palpation, will include examination of the lymph glands. This type of screening requires trained personnel. It is not generally on offer to all women as a routine check, but tends to be used for women who have discovered a breast lump by self-examination. The doctor will also check whether any breast lump is a tumour, solid in consistency, or a harmless cyst. If it is a cyst (as is commonly the case), an examination by means of a syringe will reveal this, and remove the fluid in the cyst at the same time. This is called aspiration.

The sensitivity of screening can be improved by the use of yet another method, mammography, a special X-ray technique, but this is more expensive and exposes the woman to a slight dose of radiation, with its own inherent risk.

It has been claimed that the wholesale screening of women in the high-risk category could cost an average of £5,000–£6,000 per breast cancer detected. The National Health Service is not, at present, funded for such expenditure. However, the proven success of mammographic screening programmes in the USA and Sweden has led, in Britain, to the setting up of a working group to evaluate the cost and effectiveness of a similar scheme. Screening clinics have been set up in several health districts, where women between 45 and 65 are offered annual screening, with mammograms every other year, and the effects of this on the local death rate from breast cancer are being monitored.

For anyone who can afford to pay, screening is available in private hospitals and clinics.

lung cancer

This is the commonest cancer in Britain especially in men, but now more and more frequently found in women. If the patient has a cough that brings up phlegm, cancer cells can be detected in this under the microscope. But the cancer can be detected even before these symptoms become noticeable, through the appearance of a shadow on a chest X-ray.

However, the American Cancer Society, after careful evaluation of X-ray screening, has declared it ineffective, even amongst heavy smokers. The reason was that, even though many more cases would be detected, there would be no real improvement in the rate of cure, because most types of lung cancer are notoriously difficult to cure at any stage of development. Whatever the treatment, only a small percentage of the patients is likely to survive longer than five years.

Lung cancer has an obvious, self-inflicted and avoidable cause: no detection, however early, can be as beneficial as simply not smoking at all.

cancers of the bowel (intestine)

In the case of these common cancers, it has likewise been difficult to show that any benefit would arise from the screening of a whole population. The first stage of screening bowel cancers depends on a test which detects minute invisible quantities of blood present in the faeces (bowel motions). The blood is detectable by means of paper discs impregnated with a particular chemical which reacts with the haemoglobin (red pigment) of blood. However, a positive reaction to this test does not necessarily mean that there is cancer: blood may be present in the faeces for a variety of reasons, such as benign disease, or taking aspirin. When all the patients with positive reactions have undergone further tests, only a very few will show the early stages of cancer: most of them will prove to be normally healthy, or suffering from a non-cancerous disease, such as piles. These further tests are unpleasant for the patient and are expensive and demand a lot of medical time, so this type of screening is not considered to be sufficiently rewarding.

This is bad news for those who will end up among the 17,000 people who every year die from cancer of the colon and rectum (the last sections of the bowel). Some medical authorities believe that this dismal figure can be reduced by new types of screening, aimed at those most at risk, that is, people aged 45 and over. The effectiveness of some of these tests is being evaluated.

One do-it-yourself test, now being tried out by volunteers in London, involves the use of special toilet paper which is sprayed, after use, with a chemical compound: if any blood is present, the paper will turn blue. The user will then undergo further investigations. If this test or some other tests come into general use, it should make testing for colo-rectal cancer somewhat quicker and cheaper. Most important of all, it could save many lives by allowing the disease to be detected in more people at an earlier stage.

There is a form of rare bowel cancer which has been shown to be linked to a hereditary disease, polyposis coli: polyps grow in the colon, and though not malignant in themselves, they lead to cancer, unless removed. Thus, the screening of people with a family history of polyposis could save them from developing cancer later. However, such a programme has not yet gone beyond the planning stages except for small experimental units in London.

Since there is no absolutely certain way of preventing cancer, the prompt reporting of any symptoms must be the next best line of defence, together with taking advantage of any screening that may be available.

HOW TO RECOGNISE CANCER

In their earliest beginnings, all cancers are completely symptom-less, and therefore undetectable. As they grow, they manifest themselves in a variety of ways, and there is no single symptom or physical sign that indicates with certainty the presence of a malignant growth. However, there are certain warning signs which should *never* be ignored or glossed over:

○ thickening or lump in the breast, testicles, or elsewhere
○ change in bowel or bladder habits
○ nagging cough or hoarseness
○ unusual bleeding or discharge
○ a sore that does not heal
○ obvious change in wart or mole
○ indigestion or difficulty in swallowing.

Other symptoms which should be taken seriously, especially when accompanying any of those just mentioned, are:

○ weight loss not due to any change in diet, or else due to an unexplained loss of appetite
○ pain, when it is persistent: this is not, as a rule, a symptom of early cancer, but there are some exceptions
○ undue lassitude or malaise.

For how long should you observe any of these symptoms before reporting it? The answer is, in most cases: no time at all. Symptoms such as hoarseness, coughing or pain become worry-ing only if they persist. However, even there you should not delay longer than two weeks before reporting the symptom to your doctor.

The golden rule is: do not panic, but do not waste time, and consult your doctor right away. All symptoms can indicate a benign condition. The doctor's explanation will save you unnecessary anxiety.

It is a great mistake to suppose that if you pretend to yourself that you have noticed nothing, the problem will simply go away; and just as foolish to feel embarrassed about 'bothering' your doctor, in case it all turns out to be a false alarm.

Where there is a malignant cause for the symptom, reporting it promptly is likely to make the treatment more effective, and increase the chances of success.

the common symptoms of cancer

The symptoms of the commonest cancers can be thought of as falling into the following groups:

chest and throat symptoms
They include a persistent cough: the bringing up of discoloured mucus, with or without hoarseness; shortness of breath, spitting up blood. Most of these are the familiar signs of the common cold and bronchitis; the time to take them seriously is if they appear unheralded by any cold; if they persist beyond the usual time for recovering from a cold; if they are accompanied by loss of weight or difficulty in swallowing.

These symptoms are associated with lung cancer, and various cancers of the throat, as well as with many non-malignant conditions of these organs.

abdominal symptoms
The symptoms to watch are: persistent constipation or diarrhoea or unexplained change in bowel habit; passing blood in the motions or urine; persistent indigestion, nausea or vomiting; difficulty in swallowing. In the majority of cases, their presence indicates some benign condition, but they may also be symptoms of cancer and should therefore be reported promptly, especially if there is also any weight loss.

Blood in the urine is associated with cancer of the kidneys and the bladder; blood in the bowel motions and persistent constipation or diarrhoea with cancer of the colon and rectum. Persistent indigestion and difficulty in swallowing, accompanied by loss of appetite, may be a sign of stomach or oesophageal cancer.

swellings
In this category come persistent and (usually) painless lumps under the skin, which could indicate malignant growths in the skin or in the tissues just under it. Other symptoms to take note of are dark moles which change size or shape or colour, or which become crusted or bleed; or the appearance of a new mole in adult life (over the age of 30), also a mole on the leg which starts to stick to tights. These could show the presence of malignant melanoma.

For women, lumps in the breast are important; also any changes in the shape and size of a breast, puckering or dimpling of the skin, or retraction (indrawing) of the nipple. For men, lumps in the testicles may be a danger sign, swelling or hardening is more likely than a localised lump. Another kind of swelling which women should report is swelling of the abdomen (such as occurs in pregnancy): this may indicate the presence of a harmless ovarian cyst, or of an ovarian cancer.

discharges
These include bleeding between menstrual periods; unusually heavy or irregular periods; clear or discoloured discharge from the vagina: bleeding after the menopause. These symptoms may indicate a cancer of the cervix, or of the womb lining (endometrium) or of an ovary. A discharge, or bleeding, or blood-stained discharge from a nipple may be related to breast cancer.

unlocalised symptoms
These are symptoms which cannot be ascribed to any particular part of the body, but are, rather, a sort of general malaise.

Almost everyone suffers from them at some time, for no alarming reason; but if they persist, they should certainly be reported. They include constant fatigue and lassitude, loss of appetite, weight loss, and running a temperature. There may be dozens of different reasons for them, but leukaemia and lymphoma are among the remote possibilities. Tiredness with bleeding into the skin (which looks like bruising) or from the nose, or infections that do not clear up may indicate leukaemia.

hormonal effects
Some (fairly rare) cancers have a striking effect on the body's hormone supply. Hormones are substances which are produced and released directly into the bloodstream by ductless (endocrine) glands. Among these glands are the thyroid and parathyroid (in the neck), the adrenal (above the kidneys) and the pituitary (below the brain); the pancreas, the ovaries and the testes also act as endocrine glands. The hormones they manufacture are chemical messengers, instructing other organs to develop or to function in various ways.

When a tumour (not necessarily malignant) arises in endocrine tissue, it too may secrete hormones during growth, so causing overproduction. Excess hormones released into the bloodstream will cause observable symptoms: thus cancer of the adrenal glands, which produce (amongst others) sex hormones, may cause a woman to show some male sexual characteristics, and vice versa. It should be emphasised that a man or a woman showing 'wrong' secondary sexual characteristics (for example, female facial hair) is by no means necessarily a sign of cancer.

Other endocrine cancers show other symptoms; and some tumours can change the type of hormone released, and even bring about hormone production in non-endocrine tissue.

The amount of hormone in the bloodstream can be ascertained by laboratory techniques; any excess of hormone may indicate the presence of cancer or it may just indicate a benign overaction of the normal gland.

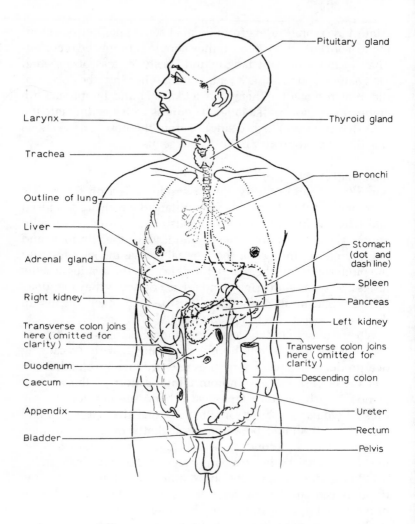

Positions of the main organs in the man.

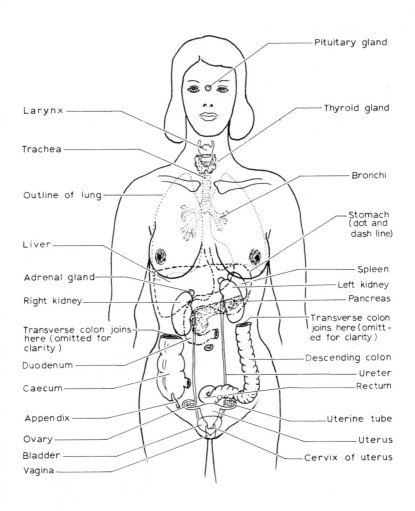

Pituitary gland

Larynx

Trachea

Outline of lung

Liver

Adrenal gland

Right kidney

Transverse colon joins here (omitted for clarity)

Duodenum

Caecum

Appendix

Ovary

Bladder

Vagina

Thyroid gland

Bronchi

Stomach (dot and dash line)

Spleen

Left kidney

Pancreas

Transverse colon joins here (omitted for clarity)

Descending colon

Ureter

Rectum

Uterine tube

Uterus

Cervix of uterus

Positions of the main organs in the woman.

go and see your doctor

It cannot be too strongly emphasised that any of these symptoms may represent non-cancerous – though possibly still serious – illnesses. A stomach ulcer produces symptoms similar to those of stomach cancer, and blood in the motions is a common symptom of piles; blood in the urine may be simply due to an infection. So, if you have any worrying symptoms, consult your GP without loss of time: if he (or she) is not immediately able to set your mind at rest, he can direct you towards further specialist investigations. Whether your complaint turns out to be cancer or not, it may still need treatment.

It is probable that after examining you, the GP may carry out initial tests himself, or send, for example, blood and urine to a laboratory for initial investigation. Alternatively, or in addition, your GP may send you to a hospital outpatients' clinic for specialist investigations.

If he does not, and you do not feel sufficiently reassured by the treatment he suggests, you have the right to request the GP to refer you to a specialist. He has the right to refuse, though he probably will not. You can complain to the Family Practitioner Committee if you do not get satisfaction, but this should not be necessary. As a last resort, a private consultation with another GP should get you the referral you want.

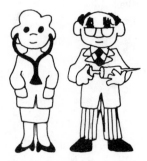

for 'he' read 'he or she'

HOW CANCER IS DIAGNOSED

The patient who has observed any of the warning signs may have some psychological obstacles to overcome. The first is the natural urge to ignore the evidence. When this has been got over, and he or she has been to see the doctor, there is often a temptation to yield to a despairing feeling of being under a sentence of death with no appeal.

This needs strongly to be resisted. Even if the diagnosis confirms one's forebodings, this need not be the end of the last chapter: there is a great deal that medical science is already able to do, and the best way in which the patient can help himself is to refuse to collapse into passivity, but rather to accept the bad news in a spirit of defiance. There is some evidence to suggest that a lowering of one's mental defences may act to lower one's physical ones: conversely, an angry refusal to surrender may bolster these defences. It will not, in itself, cause the tumour to disappear, but it may greatly reinforce whatever treatment is decided upon.

The first step: the GP's assessment

Having listened to the patient's story, the GP will carry out a routine clinical examination, in the course of which he will look for evidence of the presence of a tumour in the chest, the abdomen or any other sites that may be involved. He will inspect the lymph glands (in the armpit, chest and groin, where they may be felt) to see if they are enlarged, and ask about general symptoms, such as loss of weight, or of appetite. He may take a cervical smear for testing.

If the GP is not, at this point, able to state confidently that there is no serious disorder, he will refer the patient to the outpatients' department of a hospital for an opinion by a specialist. This may be a physician or surgeon concerned with treating the part of the body in question (for example, a chest specialist) or a cancer specialist at the oncology clinic. The GP will write to him, outlining the patient's case history and his own diagnosis, and asking him to examine the patient as soon as possible. If cancer is suspected, an appointment is likely to be arranged with only a short delay: a couple of weeks at the outside.

When the patient has undergone some form of screening, such as a cervical smear test or blood or urine test, the GP will be informed of the results in the first instance. If there is any abnormality, he will arrange a hospital referral in the same way.

the second step: the hospital clinic

The specialist takes the patient's history again, in greater detail, and also examines him again, following the pointers in the GP's letter. He then decides, on the basis of all this, what further tests are required.

blood tests

Illnesses often leave characteristic traces in the blood, which may be circumstantial or sometimes direct evidence of cancer. For the tests, a small amount of blood is taken from a vein in the patient's arm by means of a syringe. Some of this goes to the haematological laboratory, and some to the clinical chemistry laboratory.

Haematological tests can show that there is anaemia, a deficiency of red blood cells. This may mean that there has been a considerable blood loss. This is a characteristic feature of some lymphomas and leukaemias, especially when the white cells are immature in appearance, which is a feature of some types of leukaemia.

Chemical tests may reveal a disturbance in the functioning of the kidneys or the liver, and can sometimes point to cancer involving other tissues, such as bones. Occasionally, the blood is tested specifically for products such as some proteins or hormones or enzymes, which are characteristic of a particular cancer.

The results of blood tests are communicated to the GP: they are usually available within a week or so. Usually the patient will be seen again in the hospital to discuss the results.

the third step: further investigations

As a rule, blood tests in themselves are not enough for the diagnosis and full evaluation of cancer.

Cytological tests, that is, examination of cells under the microscope, can be carried out on sputum (for cancer of the bronchus), cervical smears (for cancer of the neck of the womb), on skin scrapings (for basal cell epithelioma, a skin cancer) and on gastric washings (for cancer of the stomach).

Other investigative techniques are X-rays, radioisotope scanning, magnetic-resonance scanning, CT scanning, ultrasound scanning, surgical biopsy and endoscopy. Any one or all of these may be needed to establish the exact nature and extent of a cancer.

Patients undergoing these tests often find them time-consuming and exhausting, and constant outpatient attendance at the hospital is apt to increase their natural feelings of anxiety and depression. It is sometimes better for them to be admitted to hospital, where all the tests can be done more quickly and conveniently for the patients, as well as the medical staff.

staging

The tests outlined here not only help to determine whether there is a malignant tumour, but also to find out how far it has progressed and spread, and where the metastases (if any) are. Assessing the degree of spread is called staging the cancer, from stage 1 to 4. What happens at each stage is different for each type of cancer, but, basically, in stage 1 the tumour is confined to a defined location, at stage 4 it has spread to most other parts of the body. The kind of treatment that will be chosen is likely to depend on the stage of the cancer.

X-rays

Most people have some experience of this investigative method. X-rays, a type of electromagnetic radiation, are aimed at the body: different organs vary in the amount of radiation that they allow to pass through, and the resulting pattern of shadows is recorded on photographic plates.

Bones are radio-opaque, that is, they obstruct most of the rays, and so show up as strong white shadows; they are easiest to 'visualise'. The lungs, on the other hand, let the rays pass through, being hollow: this means that any obstruction, such as a tumour, shows up as a patch of shadow on the film.

Other organs can be made to show up on film by being filled with some radio-opaque substance, or contrast medium. In order to visualise the stomach, the radiologist gives the patient, beforehand, a glassful of a barium sulphate compound to drink: this is called a barium meal (and is usually flavoured to make it acceptable). It is not digested, and when it has done its work of outlining the stomach, passes harmlessly out of the body. To visualise the bowel, barium is administered via the anus (barium enema). Intermediate parts of the digestive system can be visualised by observing the passage of the barium through them over a period of hours.

For the kidneys, the ureter and the bladder, the contrast medium is an iodine compound, injected into a vein and observed as it passes into the kidneys and thence through vessels called ureters into the bladder. This method is called intravenous pyelography (IVP) or intravenous urography (IVU), and reveals kidney malfunctions and obstructions in the urinary system.

Different radio-opaque contrast media are also used to examine the blood vessels for signs of obstruction, such as might be caused by a tumour; also to examine the lymphatic system (lymphangiogram) and the spine (myelogram). The spinal cord is sometimes affected by primary and secondary cancers. For treatment, it is vital to pinpoint precisely the position of any growth or suspected growth. A contrast dye is injected into the fluid-filled space surrounding the spinal cord by a needle inserted between two lumbar vertebrae at the bottom of the back (i.e. a lumbar puncture). This is sometimes uncomfortable but not dangerous. Normally the dye flows freely around the cord and any impediment to this flow indicates a precise level for a suspected growth.

CT scanning

CT scanning (computer-axial tomography) is a new refinement: by means of special equipment, multiple X-rays are taken all round a part of the body, and the information obtained from all of them is combined by a computer to build up an image or cross-section of the whole organ. This technique can give valuable information. It was used mainly to investigate the inside of the head, but is now used for the whole body. In some hospital units it is replacing IVP.

Though these X-ray procedures are tedious and occasionally unpleasant for the patient, they represent the least painful and dangerous way of examining many areas of the body.

radio-isotope scanning

Some tissues of the body attract certain chemicals: for instance, the thyroid gland takes up all the iodine in the body, and bone takes up phosphate. When such chemicals are administered in their radioactive form, the result is radioactive emission from the tissues so that they can be seen as an image on a television screen or on photographic film, and any abnormality in these tissues is shown up. The radioactive isotopes of various chemicals are used to scan the liver, the bones and some other organs. The amounts of radioactivity are too minuscule to do harm, and the tests are usually easier for the patient than many of the X-ray procedures.

ultrasonography

This is scanning by inaudible high-frequency sound waves (ultrasound). A microphone-like instrument is passed over the surface of the body: this probe beams out sound waves and picks up the returning echoes, which are used to build up an image of the internal organs. The echo pattern, reproduced on a TV screen (which can be photographed to make a permanent record) can show the location of tumours and give much useful information about the abdominal cavity, especially the liver.

For the patient, this is the easiest method: it is painless and demands only the ability to sit or lie still while the test is done.

nuclear magnetic-resonance scanning (NMR)
This is a sophisticated new scanning technique, available in only a few hospitals at the moment, which uses a combination of electric and magnetic fields to measure the water content of the tissues being examined. Cancer growths usually have a different water content from the normal tissues amongst which they grow, and so return a different signal, which the scanner picks up and uses to build up an image of the tumour. Magnetic resonance scanning is a painless way of investigating tissues not accessible to other forms of scanning and, so far as is known, carries no risks to the patient.

endoscopy
This is the general name for the technique of directly looking into internal organs by means of optical instruments: these usually take the form of lighted tubes which may be rigid or flexible, and equipped with lenses or optical fibres (which permit seeing round bends). They are passed into the body through one of its natural openings: the mouth, the nose, the urethra, the rectum. There is an appropriate instrument for each. A sigmoidoscope and a colonoscope are used to examine the bowel; a colposcope is used for the uterine cervix and a cystoscope for the bladder. For the upper digestive tract, including the stomach, a gastro-scope is used; for the lungs, a bronchoscope.

Endoscopy may be uncomfortable, but is seldom painful: the patients may be given a sedative, to make them feel more relaxed or comfortable, or even a light anaesthetic.

biopsy
This test is used to confirm beyond doubt the presence of a cancer, and is essential for determining the appropriate treat-ment. It involves the removal of a sample of the suspect tissue, and its examination under a microscope.

Samples of tissue are obtained in various ways depending on where it is, and usually under a local anaesthetic. In the case of skin, a scalpel is used to detach a tiny fragment of it. For many internal organs, a hollow needle is inserted into the body to extract a minute amount of tissue. Such needle biopsy is also used to determine the nature of breast lumps if they are thought to be cysts.

When a cervical smear test shows the presence of abnormal cells, a cone biopsy, the removal of a conical fragment of tissue, is usually done. This may be all the treatment necessary for small early cervix tumours.

Sometimes a biopsy is combined with endoscopy, by using an instrument designed to take a tissue sample in the course of the visual examination. When a cervical smear test shows the presence of abnormal cells, a colposcopic examination is usually done. At this examination, any suspicious areas can be biopsied. Following this, the suspect area can in many cases be treated with a laser beam which vaporises the abnormal tissue. The treated area rapidly heals to normal cervical epithelium.

surgical biopsy
In cases where the location of a tumour is known but there is some uncertainty about its nature, a biopsy may be performed under general anaesthesia. Typically, in the case of a large breast tumour, the lump is removed, and a section of it is immediately frozen and processed by a pathologist who reports back to the surgeon, usually within half an hour, while the patient remains anaesthetised. If the tumour is found to be malignant, the surgeon goes on, there and then, to take whatever surgical measures are necessary. This saves the patient from having to undergo two separate operations. However, it should only be done if the patient's consent has been obtained beforehand to those other measures.

It is thought that there might be a slight risk of locally spreading the cancer where scalpels or needles are used in a biopsy. But the risk inherent in not carrying out a biopsy is generally very much greater.

bone marrow examination
The bone marrow is richly perfused by the blood and any cancer that gets into the bloodstream can potentially go to the marrow.

Thus sampling the bone marrow is part of the routine staging for some cancers, especially cancers of the blood and the lymph glands (leukaemias and lymphomas). The marrow is taken from the hip bone or breast bone under local anaesthetic: a wide needle is inserted through the bone into the marrow cavity and a small amount of marrow is sucked out with a syringe. This is momentarily painful.

THE TREATMENT OF CANCER

In setting out to cure cancer, the chief types of treatment available are surgery, radiotherapy, chemotherapy and hormone therapy. The first two are local and work by removing or destroying the cancerous tissue in the body. The third and fourth are systemic and affect the whole body. Hormone therapy works by altering hormonal influence on tumours. These techniques are not mutually exclusive, and the treatment of a malignant tumour may involve more than one of them.

surgery

This is the classic cancer treatment and, until early this century, used to be the only one available. It is probably the first treatment that occurs to the lay person, but it is by no means a universal cure-all, and can be used only in certain strictly defined circumstances.

when a cancer is operable

First, the cancer must not be growing in a vital tissue, one that is needed to sustain life, and which cannot be removed completely without killing the patient: for example, the brain or the liver.

Secondly, the cancer must be localised, that is, restricted to the site of origin. An operation will not cure if the cancer has already invaded distant tissues through the blood or lymphatic circulations, or if it has spread to adjacent organs, especially if these are vital organs. Nor will an operation do much good if, as in the case of lymphomas and leukaemias, the cancer has actually arisen in the blood or lymph vessels, and is by its very nature present in all parts of the body. However, surgery may be useful in relieving symptoms (for example a bowel blockage) even if the cancer has spread, or in removing as much tumour as possible before giving radiotherapy or chemotherapy.

Thirdly, a patient cannot undergo surgery if he is too weak – either because of the cancer, or because of some other condition – to have a good chance of surviving the operation.

A most important factor in deciding whether to operate must be the patient's own attitude. An operation may involve a degree of mutilation or disablement, and the patient may feel that life on those terms is not worth living, and may demand some other treatment – or none. In any case, the question of carrying out any surgical procedure without the patient's consent should not arise.

The surgeon cannot always be sure, until he has begun to operate, what the operation will involve. He should discuss the matter with the patient beforehand and obtain his or her signed consent to any surgical measures that may be found necessary. If the patient refuses to give a carte-blanche of this sort, two operations may be necessary, the first one being merely exploratory. This is much harder on the patient and may be more dangerous, which is why the surgeon will probably be against the idea, and will want to combine exploration and treatment in one operation. The patient however has a choice, and should not be prevented from exercising it. Psychologically, it may be better to choose what is right for him or her, rather than having choices imposed.

breast tumour operation
The technique of surgical biopsy has already been described. The patient waits, anaesthetised, while laboratory tests are performed on a frozen section of suspect tissue: the results decide how extensive the operation is to be.

This procedure is often used in the case of a breast lump whose nature the surgeon is not sure about. If the tests show that it is a benign tumour, then all he needs to do is to remove it. If it is cancerous, he must decide whether to perform a lumpectomy (removal of the tumour, plus some of the surrounding tissue) or a mastectomy (removal of the whole breast); he may also remove the adjacent axillary lymph nodes.

If a surgeon is going to do a frozen section biopsy and then proceed, he should have decided with the patient, before the operation, whether to do a lumpectomy or mastectomy. The questions a patient may wish to ask include: if I have a lumpectomy instead of a mastectomy, what difference will this make to my life expectancy? What are the possibilities of reconstructing a breast? Can a nipple be left at the original operation? What about the side effects from removing the lymph nodes (such as painful swollen arm and susceptibility to local infection which occurs after radical surgery)? What causes this and how important is it to have the lymph nodes removed?

some other types of operation
Operations for the removal of breast tumours (which are comparatively simple to explain) are only one example of cancer surgery. But tumours arising in almost any of the organs may be suitable for surgical removal. There are very many possible operations, each with its own risks and chances of succeeding, both in removing the tumour and helping to prevent a recurrence.

Each operation is likely to involve a certain amount of physical impairment, and the patient should insist on knowing what this will be, and what difficulties he or she will face in learning to live with it.

Most people willingly accept the prospect of a simple operation scar, which will fade in time and is usually covered with clothing. But any operation that threatens to reduce a person's physical integrity in some obvious way is bound to cause distress. The removal of a skin cancer on the face, for instance, may leave a scar more conspicuous than the results of a mastectomy. The patient should ask to be told whether any other treatments – such as radiotherapy – could be used instead, and whether any corrective treatment, such as skin grafting, will be needed.

'ostomy' operations

There are procedures in which a part or whole of the body's waste disposal system – the bowel or bladder – is removed, and the body's waste products are made to discharge through a *stoma*, an artificial opening on the surface of the abdomen. When the bladder is removed, this is called a urostomy; when some or all of the ileum or the colon is removed, this is called an ileostomy, or colostomy. Ostomy operations are used not only for bowel cancer, but also for non-malignant conditions such as ulcerative colitis. In some cases, a colostomy is temporary (and can be closed later after a further operation has been done) but in most cases it is permanent. All these operations require the use of a special appliance or bag, and the learning of a special technique for its use. The prospect of it may cause considerable distress.

The mutilation can cause damaging feelings of depression or self-disgust on the part of the patient, and thus might affect sexual relationships, particularly if the healthy partner feels some repulsion. Counselling may be very effective in helping both partners to accept the disability.

Specialised organisations exist to help people who have had to undergo a mastectomy, an ostomy, or some other kinds of surgery.

However, patients should be assured that such an operation would never be done without their consent. If a surgeon suspects that it might be necessary he should warn the patient of this and explain fully how the resulting disablement is likely to affect his future life. No one should have to be afraid that he or she will wake up after an operation to discover that something he cannot accept has been done to him.

advances in surgery

An advance has been the replacement of some conventional surgical procedures by laser treatment. Laser beams can be focused with extreme accuracy to destroy tumour tissue in delicate areas, such as the brain and the spine, where conventional surgery can be hazardous and traumatic to the patient. Laser surgery is also being used in the treatment of cervical cancer. The precision is such that the surrounding healthy tissue is not damaged.

A new development in orthopaedic surgery is the replacement of cancerous sections of arm or leg bone by metal sections, so saving the limb from amputation.

after the operation

In the course of operating, the surgeon may carry out biopsies in distant tissues, so that they can be checked for signs of invasion. All the tissue that was removed in the operation undergoes tests to find out the exact nature of the tumour; if malignant, whether it is of the rapidly invasive sort, and, if so, how far it is likely to have spread. There are several possibilities:

○ The tumour is confirmed as benign and there is no cancer; there may be no need for further hospital treatment, and only a short-period monitoring of the patient's recovery. Such a follow-up is usually done in the hospital's outpatients' clinic.

○ The tumour is confirmed as malignant, but seems to be completely localised. All of it has been removed, and there are no indications that it has spread (other tests, such as X-rays, may have to be done to confirm this). It is possible that no other treatment will be needed, but the surgeon must make quite sure, and must watch out for any recurrence of the disease, and so should the patient.

○ In the case of breast cancer, for example, it is known from experience that there may be a chance of metastasis, so further therapy may be considered. The patient will have to have check-ups at the outpatients' clinic for some months, or even years.

○ The tumour is confirmed as malignant, and it is found, either during the operation or through subsequent tests, that the cancer is now growing in sites other than the site of origin and further treatment is appropriate.

further treatment

The surgeon usually consults other specialists: a radiotherapist, a medical oncologist, and sometimes a haematologist (specialist in diseases of the blood). The joint consultation regarding what would be best for the patient should take place before any treatment is started. The decision about further treatment will depend on the nature of the cancer, the degree to which it seems to have spread, the patient's condition and his attitude: in short, on all the factors which may make it necessary to resort to some treatment other than surgery.

The decision will be different for each individual patient. In many cases, even when the cancer is widespread and considerably advanced, there are treatments which can dramatically improve the patient's condition, and maintain this improvement for a long time. Sometimes a cure may be possible. However, some cancers tend to resist all the therapies currently available, and then the patient's attitude can be the most important factor in deciding on treatment. All medical treatments of cancer, whether radiotherapeutic or chemotherapeutic (drug-based) cause side-effects to a greater or lesser degree, and the patient must be the one to decide whether the benefits of a treatment outweigh its disadvantages to him.

This is inevitably a difficult decision, and nobody should allow himself to be subjected to treatment which may be time-consuming, exacting and possibly debilitating, without asking for a full explanation of it and the reasons for it, in language a lay person can understand.

radiotherapy

This technique came into use early in this century. Following the discovery by Roentgen (in 1895) of a type of electromagnetic radiation he named X-rays, it was found that these rays could, if delivered at sufficient intensity, damage living tissue; when aimed at tumours, X-rays could reduce or even destroy them.

Low-energy radiation was effective on superficial cancers, for example, of the skin, while high-energy radiation could reach deep-seated tumours. Later, other types of radiation came to be used in cancer therapy: that emitted by the radioactive element radium, and radiations produced by the radioactive isotopes of other elements, such as caesium, cobalt and iridium.

Radiotherapy is used in cancer treatment for two purposes: curative and palliative.

curative radiotherapy

The aim of this is to destroy tumour tissue. It may be used as a follow-up to surgery, to destroy any cancer cells that may still remain after the removal of a tumour. Sometimes it is used before surgery, in order to shrink tumours, making them easier to remove; or it can stand on its own as the initial treatment. A large number of specific cancers are curable by radiotherapy alone, such as cancer of the larynx and some skin cancers. Its special usefulness is in the case of cancers which cannot be surgically removed, because they are sited in vital organs; or because they are too deep-seated (as in the brain) to be accessible; or because they are widespread (as in the case of Hodgkin's disease and other lymphomas). However, radiotherapy has many other applications, as in cancers of the breast; gynaecological cancers (of the ovaries, the cervix and the womb generally); malignant tumours of the head and neck region.

Some tissues, such as the lungs, gonads (that is testes and ovaries), spinal cord and kidneys, are particularly vulnerable to the damaging effects of X-rays. Where they are normal and healthy, they should be shielded from radiation, and care must be taken in treating cancers adjacent to them.

palliative radiotherapy

The aim is to improve the quality of the patient's life by relieving the symptoms of cancer. The therapy may be used as an adjunct to other treatment, but its particular usefulness is in cases where no cure can be hoped for. Radiotherapy can relieve symptoms such as pain, bleeding, compression of nerves. It can prevent complications which sometimes accompany the extensive growth of a tumour, such a bone fracture or ulceration of the skin. Because the patient's comfort is the chief consideration, the amount of radiation applied is likely to be as low as possible, in order to minimise the risk of side-effects such as nausea.

methods used in radiotherapy

Radiation therapy can be applied in the following ways:

○ By inserting hollow tubes containing radioactive compounds into one of the body cavities. The commonest application of this is in the treatment of cervical cancer, where such a tube is inserted into the cavity of the womb and into the vagina against the neck of the womb, to irradiate the neck of the womb.

○ By implanting fine radioactive needles (for example, of iridium or caesium) into the tissue of easily accessible cancers, such as those of the mouth, and, sometimes, the breast.

In both the above applications, the diseased tissue can be thoroughly irradiated with minimal damage to the surrounding healthy tissue.

○ The commonest way of treating both superficial and deep-seated cancer is by external irradiation: X-ray therapy. Doses of radiation, measured in units called rads or grays (one gray is 100 rads), are carefully calculated by physicists, allowing radiotherapists to know precisely how much radiation is being delivered to the tumour and to the surrounding healthy tissues.

Sometimes the X-rays are beamed on to the tumour from several angles or positions simultaneously, or the X-ray beam is rotated round the patient, which allows a high dose of radiation to be focused on the cancer, while doing minimal harm to normal tissue. In some treatments, external irradiation is used initially followed by internal irradiation from radioactive implants.

The radiotherapist begins by examining the patient clinically, possibly supplemented by means of investigative X-rays, to establish the site and size of the tumour. The area to be irradiated is marked on the patient's skin. The radiotherapist works out in advance the total amount of irradiation a tumour will require, and into how many doses or fractions it is to be divided. Fractionation of X-ray doses is not only safer for the patient, but also more efficient, because tumours respond better to repeated small doses than to one large one.

The X-ray fractions are usually given daily for several days or even weeks (depending on the nature and site of the tumour), sometimes with intervals of no treatment. The actual treatment is administered by a trained radiographer. It is painless; all the patient has to do is to lie still for a few minutes. There is absolutely no risk that the treatment will make him radioactive.

radiations other than X-rays

Other types of radiation used in radiotherapy include electrons of high energy, protons, neutrons and pi-mesons. The special properties of these radiations offer better chances of curing certain types of cancer. Neutron therapy to destroy tumours works in the same way as X-ray therapy, but may be more efficient in some cases – for instance, in treating the body's soft tissues, which absorb neutrons more readily than X-rays. At present, the value of such therapy is not yet established.

Radioactive isotopes are also sometimes used systemically in radiotherapy, for example, radioactive iodine for the treatment of cancer of the thyroid gland.

side-effects of X-ray therapy

X-rays are aimed as precisely as possible to concentrate their energy on the tumour, but (unless the cancer is in the skin) to get to it they must pass through healthy tissue, and since radiation affects all living tissue, some side-effects may result. These generally disappear after the completion of the treatment.

The commonest side-effect is a feeling of nausea or tiredness, which may be accompanied by depression. In the case of X-ray treatment for skin cancers, the side-effects are soreness and reddening of the skin, like sunburn, very rarely there may be dilated blood vessels in the skin and possibly scarring (but no systemic side-effects such as nausea).

Irradiation of the digestive organs may produce disturbances, such as diarrhoea or nausea. In the case of irradiation of the head, the hair may fall out, partially or totally, if the whole head is being irradiated. This is very distressing, especially to a woman, but the hair generally grows back once treatment is over. Getting a wig before treatment helps to reduce the emotional stress.

The reduction of the patient's resistance to infection is a possible side-effect, when bones such as the spine and breastbone have to be exposed to radiation. They contain a large proportion of the body's bone marrow, in which the cellular components of the blood – platelets, red cells and white cells – are produced. The latter play an important part in destroying invading bacteria, but are easily damaged by radiation, so depriving the body of its natural defence against infection. For this reason, patients who receive radiotherapy have their blood count (the proportions of the various components) regularly checked, to make sure that the white cells are holding their own.

Intensive radiation can lead to decalcification of bones with the risk of fractures.

chemotherapy

This is the name given to the treatment of cancer by drugs, mainly chemical compounds called cytotoxic (literally, cell-poisoning) drugs, which have the ability to destroy living cells. They can cause the regression of tumours and can sometimes clear them up completely.

Chemotherapy is used in two situations: as the main treatment in advanced disease, and as an adjuvant to other therapies to help bring about a relapse-free survival.

Whilst surgery and radiotherapy are both local therapies, which are applied to particular areas of the body, chemotherapy is systemic: its effects are felt throughout the whole system. The great virtue of chemotherapy is that it can be used against widely disseminated cancers which have produced metastases throughout the body. The drawback is that cytotoxic drugs are not selective enough and do not discriminate between cancer and non-cancer cells, and can therefore produce unpleasant side-effects because of damage to normal tissues.

adjuvant chemotherapy

As well as being used to treat widespread cancer, cytotoxic drugs are being used increasingly early in the disease, to improve the control of localised cancer, and to prevent, or at least delay as much as possible, metastasis (the onset of secondary deposits in other parts of the body).

This approach is being tried out for several common cancers, notably breast cancer, whose response to treatment is notoriously unpredictable: it has a tendency to reappear at sites distant from the breast – bones, lungs, liver and sometimes the brain – long after the local breast tumour has apparently been eradicated. It is not yet established whether the ultimate benefits to the patient of this treatment are such as to outweigh its often distressing side-effects.

how chemotherapy began

Chemotherapy destroys cancer cells by interfering in some way with their ability to reproduce themselves. Its inauspicious origins lie in the development of poison gas for use in warfare. One of these, mustard gas, was discovered to kill white blood cells. This gave scientists the notion of using a similar compound to treat cancers characterised by white-cell overproduction, such as lymphomas and leukaemias. Although this drug was temporary in its effects and too toxic to be used, it was found that, by chemical modification of it, drugs could be produced that would kill tumour cells without killing or permanently damaging the patient. Once the tumour was destroyed, the damaged normal cells would recover.

Subsequently, many other cytotoxic compounds have been developed and used in clinical practice; there are now more than 40 of them.

how chemotherapy is administered
Some drugs are given by mouth, and others by injection. Yet other drugs are administered by means of an intravenous drip; there is little or no discomfort from this method. The length of the treatment depends on the response to it. Often it is given in stages or 'pulses', with breaks of three or four weeks in between, to give the normal cells, which tend to recover faster than the cancer ones, a chance to re-establish themselves.

making the most of cytotoxic drugs

Cytotoxic therapy must be designed to do the least possible damage to the patient. How is this aim to be achieved with drugs which are not selective in their effects?

One way is to use several drugs – up to three or four – in the course of a treatment, each one having a different action: the combination has a greater effect on the tumour than any one drug on its own. Moreover, each drug has a different effect on normal tissues. For instance, a drug which is toxic to the bone marrow may not be toxic to the gastro-intestinal tract, so that giving several drugs in smaller doses together instead of a single drug in a large single dose, may limit each type of side-effect.

Diseases such as Hodgkin's disease (a cancer of the lymph glands) and testicular seminoma, which were not curable with individual drug therapy, are now routinely cured with cytotoxic combinations.

side-effects of cytotoxic drugs

The effect of cytotoxic drugs on normal tissues varies enormously. Those drugs which work by disrupting the cells' reproductive process do most damage to rapidly reproducing cells. This makes them effective in destroying tumours, but also harmful to normal rapidly multiplying cells, such as those of bone marrow, of the hair follicles, of the lining of the digestive tract and of the testes.

The amount of a drug that can safely be given is limited by its effect on the bone marrow, the source of the blood cells. Excessive damage to the marrow can cause death, either from bleeding, when the cells which produce blood platelets are damaged, or from infection, when the white blood cells are destroyed. Specific blood transfusions can be used to counter these effects.

The effect on the hair follicles is to make the hair fall out: not only on the head, but sometimes also eyebrows, eyelashes and also body hair. This is deeply distressing to patients: for some, it is the most feared and resented side of cancer chemotherapy. Losing one's hair is a severe blow to the morale, even though it is not important in terms of physical health (and eventually the hair will grow again, though not necessarily the same colour or texture as before). Women faced with the prospect of chemotherapy should provide themselves with an attractive wig.

Another important side-effect of cytotoxic drugs is disturbance of the digestive system, resulting in nausea and vomiting. This may be due to the damage these drugs do to the cells of the lining of the intestines, or else to their effect on chemical receptors in the brain. Patients who have endured successive periods of drug treatment, and have had repeated experience of these unpleasant symptoms, may find that this has induced 'conditioned vomiting', in which the patient vomits in the mere expectation of receiving the drug. Here, as in the case of hair loss, cancer therapy is seen to have a psychological as well as a physiological aspect. But nowadays drugs to prevent vomiting are given before treatment and advice is given as to diet.

There are other unwelcome side-effects: tiredness and depression, diarrhoea, skin rashes and soreness; there may also be a loss of fertility. In women, fertility usually returns when the treatment ends, but a man may become permanently sterile.

what is being done about side-effects?

Less noxious compounds are being developed. These are modified versions of well-tested cytotoxic drugs, with reduced side-effects, while still efficacious against tumours. They are increasingly used where it is not cure but palliation of the effects of cancer that is hoped for.

Specific antidotes are being developed. These allow certain cytotoxic drugs to be used in very high doses to destroy a large number of cancer cells: the antidote, appropriately timed, 'rescues' normal cells from permanent harm. It is not known exactly why normal cells are easier to rescue than diseased ones, but this has not prevented doctors from exploiting this advantage in particular cancers.

It is impossible to do away with side-effects altogether, but as chemotherapy becomes more widely used and more sophisticated, new ways of coping are being developed.

Where chemotherapy is not prolonging life significantly and the side-effects are extremely distressing, the patient should be allowed to decide whether the treatment is to be continued.

hormone therapy

Like chemotherapy, hormone therapy may involve the giving of a chemical compound, but its aim is rather different: to destroy the tumour by cutting its lifeline.

Hormones are substances produced by the endocrine glands and transmitted by the blood circulation to control the functions of distant organs. They are responsible for the growth and maintenance of many tissues, in particular the sex organs both of men and women. Hormone-dependent organs in women include the breasts and the womb, controlled by female hormones such as oestrogen and progesterone; in men the prostate gland is governed by male hormones (androgens) such as testosterone.

Cancers arising from these organs often retain many characteristics of the tissue of origin, including being dependent on the supply of hormones to maintain growth. This dependency has been exploited by doctors in various ways, to block and even reverse the growth of tumours, particularly in the breast and the prostate.

Breast cancer, even when advanced, can often be controlled for as long as several years by means of hormone therapy. The first line of defence is the reduction of the tumour's oestrogen supply. Because of its effectiveness and lack of side-effects, the most popular method in recent years for pre-menopausal women has been the use of an anti-hormone, such as tamoxifen, which blocks the take-up by the cancer cells of the oestrogen in the circulation. This may bring about regression of even widespread cancer.

The problem with breast cancer, however, is that the regression may be only temporary: it tends to recur and to metastasise in the bones and elsewhere, and further measures may be necessary.

Another approach is to cut off the oestrogen supply by removing or rendering inactive the ovaries, which produce it. This may be achieved by chemotherapy or by radiotherapy, or by an operation (oophorectomy), sometimes done at the same time as the removal of the original breast tumour, as a preventive measure against recurrence. Or this operation may be kept in reserve as a further measure should the tumour recur.

Other hormones, such as testosterone and progesterone, may be administered to counter the action of oestrogen.

In the analogous case of the prostate, advanced cancer can be profoundly influenced by giving oestrogen and other hormones, and also anti-hormones, to block the supply of testosterone. The testes, which produce it, may be rendered inactive by removal (orchidectomy) or by chemotherapy.

The side-effects of hormone therapy may be masculinising or feminising.

Cancer of the lining of the womb is also in many cases responsive to hormonal treatment.

However, not all cancers of the sex organs are of hormone-dependent kind; those which are not, do not respond to hormone therapy. Much research is being devoted, at present, to finding methods of assessing accurately the hormone profile of individual cancer cells, in order to identify precisely which patients are most likely to respond. It remains to be established whether such subtle biochemical methods can be applied to other kinds of cancers. These must presumably possess their own growth factors, equivalent to hormones, and when these have been identified, methods can perhaps be found of blocking their action.

choosing the best treatment

A great many different types of cancer have been identified. Given the variety of therapies available, and the fact that patients with apparently identical tumours may respond in quite different ways to the same therapy, a whole volume could be filled with the detailed description of the treatments for any one cancer. However, it is possible to outline the reasoning behind the decision to adopt one or another method, or a combination of several.

In the best circumstances, surgery alone may be enough to cure a patient: given such an assurance, the patient will probably think that the pain or discomfort that goes with a major operation is a reasonable price to pay. The price may still be acceptable even when it includes mutilation, such as losing a breast or a limb; or the loss of fertility, as when the testicles or ovaries are removed.

However, surgery may be inadequate or even counter-productive, when:

○ the removal of a tumour would endanger the patient's life, or make it not worth living;
○ the cancer has spread widely;
○ when it is, by its very nature, growing in many parts of the body;
○ it has a high chance of reappearing in other tissues in spite of apparently complete surgical removal.

In the first three cases, the surgeon may carry out biopsies to confirm the diagnosis, but the actual treatment will be left to the oncologist, who may treat the cancer with radiation, drugs, hormones, or some combination, in sequence, of any of these. When undergoing radiotherapy and chemotherapy, the patient must pay the further price of side-effects which may be distressing.

In the fourth case, the decision is rather more complicated. Though no one who is treated surgically for cancer can be guaranteed a cure, in many cases it is possible to assure a patient that the chances of recurrence are so remote that they can be discounted. But there are some localised cancers, notably breast cancer, for which this assurance cannot be given, because they have a propensity to come back – in adjacent or distant sites.

The techniques which are used to prevent a 'distant relapse' are adjuvant treatments, on the principle that techniques found to be effective in the treatment of established advanced disease could be equally valuable in prevention.

The arguments against adjuvant treatment are that:

○ not all the people who have had localised treatment are actually at risk of a distant relapse
○ adjuvant treatment is at best a nuisance for the patient, and at worst may produce extremely unpleasant toxic side-effects.

Nevertheless, it is becoming clear that adjuvant treatment, though sometimes unpleasant, can be effective in preventing or delaying relapse.

follow-up after therapy

Even when treatment appears to have succeeded completely, patients will be asked to come back to be examined for any signs of recurrence, and may be followed up for several years – at gradually lengthening intervals.

CURE AND REMISSION

Because of the nature of cancer, it is never possible for the doctors to say that every single cancer cell has been eliminated. This makes it difficult to say categorically that anyone has been cured. Cure in cancer means that the individual who has been treated will have as good a chance of surviving to a ripe old age as he would have had, had the cancer never occurred, and then dying of something else. Given that the proof of cure may not become available for many years, the effectiveness of treatment is measured by the relapse-free period following treatment.

A five-year 'cure' rate for a type of cancer means that if the patient survives free of symptoms for five years, there is unlikely to be a recurrence – not that he will die after five years. The number of years varies with each cancer: for some kinds, a two year symptom-free period is enough to assume that a recurrence is unlikely; for others, five, ten or more years.

Cancer statistics also deal with the concept of a 'survival rate': the percentage of sufferers from any type of cancer who survive a specific number of years (one, three or five) after treatment. The chances of surviving five years depends on the type of cancer – from 10% for lung cancer to over 50% for cancer of the bladder, for example.

The complete disappearance of symptoms for a time may be a cure, or a remission. Doctors talk of complete remission when no tumour can be found anywhere and all the symptoms have disappeared – only time will then tell whether the patient is 'cured'. Partial remission means that the tumour has been substantially reduced in size. What distinguishes a complete remission from a cure, is that the tumour eventually returns. So, occasionally remissions may prove to be cures, and hoped-for cures may turn out to be remissions. When an elderly patient is enabled by a remission to live out something like the term of his natural life, the distinction becomes less meaningful.

when is a cancer considered incurable?

The simplest answer is: when it has become so widely disseminated that no form of therapy can hope to eliminate it completely. The point of incurability will be different for different types of tumour: some spread so rapidly, that the presence of metastases can be taken for granted from an early stage.

'Incurable' does not mean the same as 'untreatable', nor yet 'terminal'. To some people, incurable cancer means only one thing: rapid and agonised progression to the grave. This fearful prospect is by no means inevitable or even usual. People with incurable cancer may still be given treatment to prolong their useful lives, sometimes for years. It is only when all therapeutic measures have been exhausted, that the terminal stage is reached, at which point all that can be done is to make the last days easier.

some common types of cancer

CANCER SITE	Some Established Causes	Metastatic Sites	Early Symptoms*	Advanced Symptoms*	Treatment	Five-Year Survival Rate‡	Comments
Bladder	smoking occupational factors such as dyes	liver bones lung lymph nodes	blood in urine	more frequent urination pain in lower abdomen	surgery radiotherapy chemotherapy	50%	
Blood acute lymphatic leukaemia	ionising radiation	lymph nodes bone marrow	susceptibility to infections lassitude bruising	fever swelling of lymph nodes bone pain	chemotherapy	60% + in children (poorer in adults)	occurs chiefly in children
chronic lymphatic leukaemia		lymph nodes bone marrow	as above	as above	chemotherapy radiotherapy	30–40%	
acute myeloid leukaemia		lymph nodes bone marrow	as above	as above	chemotherapy radiotherapy	20%	
chronic myeloid leukaemia		lymph nodes bone marrow	as above	as above	chemotherapy radiotherapy	less than 20%	

Bone	may be caused by radiation	lungs		pain fever swelling	surgery radiotherapy adjuvant chemo-therapy	20–30%	
Brain			persistent headache, fits, sensory changes	impaired movement, speech, vision, memory	surgery radiotherapy chemotherapy	10%	rare as primary cancer
Breast	some hereditary influence hormone influence early menarche plus late or no child-bearing	bone lung liver lymph nodes skin	breast lump (generally painless)	dimpling of skin retraction of nipple discharge from nipple	mastectomy lumpectomy radiotherapy adjuvant chemo-therapy oophorectomy adrenalectomy hormone therapy	50–60%	risk of recurrence remains even after 5 years

Continued

* ‡ See notes on page 95

CANCER SITE	Some Established Causes	Metastatic Sites	Early Symptoms*	Advanced Symptoms*	Treatment	Five-Year Survival Rate‡	Comments
Cervix uteri (neck of womb)	may be associated with genital virus many partners	lung lymph nodes	bleeding between periods and after menopause	vaginal bleeding after intercourse vaginal discharge	surgery radiotherapy	more than 50%	may be discovered at cervical smear check-up
Colon (large intestine, large bowel) and rectum	may be dietary	liver lung lymph nodes	change in bowel habits	persistent constipation bleeding from rectum anaemia pain in lower abdomen	surgery radiotherapy chemotherapy (least successful)	30%	
Kidney (and other urinary organs)	occupational	lymph nodes lung bone	blood in urine	local pain fever pain in side lump in side	surgery radiotherapy	35%	

Larynx (voice box)	smoking a strong factor	lymph nodes lung	persistent hoarseness	sore throat pain in ear	radiotherapy surgery	55–60%	
Liver and bile ducts	hepatitis B connection with cirrhosis	lymph nodes		lassitude loss of weight and appetite abdominal pain	surgery chemotherapy	1–4%	rare as primary cancer in the UK
Lung	smoking occupational factors (asbestos)	bone liver brain lymph nodes adrenal glands bone marrow	chronic cough chest infection shortness of breath blood in sputum	hoarseness chest pains weight loss difficulty in swallowing	surgery radiotherapy chemotherapy	less than 10%	accounts for 30% of all cancer in men and 8% in women in UK

* ‡ See notes on page 95

Continued

CANCER SITE	Some Established Causes	Metastatic Sites	Early Symptoms*	Advanced Symptoms*	Treatment	Five-Year Survival Rate‡	Comments
Lymphatic system Hodgkin's disease		spleen bone marrow bone, liver, lungs	persistent painless swelling of lymph nodes	lassitude fever weight loss	radiotherapy chemotherapy surgery	80% in children, 60% in adults	
non-Hodgkin's lymphoma	possibly viral	liver, bone, bone marrow brain lungs	as above	as above	radiotherapy chemotherapy surgery	35%	
Oesophagus (gullet)	dietary factors alcohol (especially if smoking)	lymph nodes lung liver	difficulty in swallowing	chest or back pain weight loss	surgery radiotherapy	less than 10%	

Ovary	hormonal	liver lymph nodes	abdominal swelling (ascites)	ascites (accumulation of fluid in abdominal cavity) abdominal pain	surgery radiotherapy adjuvant chemo-therapy	25%	benign cysts may give similar symptoms
Pancreas		lymph nodes lung liver	irregularity of bowel action some weight loss	abdominal pain jaundice weight loss	surgery radiotherapy (palliative only)	less than 5%	
Prostate		lymph nodes bone	difficulty in urinating	more frequent urination pain	radiotherapy surgery hormone therapy	35%	

* ‡ See notes on page 95

Continued

CANCER SITE	Some Established Causes	Metastatic Sites	Early Symptoms*	Advanced Symptoms*	Treatment	Five-Year Survival Rate‡	Comments
Skin malignant melanoma	UV radiation	lymph nodes brain lung liver (highly invasive)	itch in mole; change in size, colour or shape of brown mole; new brown mole in an adult inflammation around a mole	crusting or bleeding of a mole; appearance of lump in previously flat pigmented mole; new pigmented spots coming up around a mole	surgery radiotherapy	50–60% (90% if observed early)	
other skin cancers	UV radiation occupational	lymph nodes (not very invasive)	painless lump or nodule scaliness of skin bleeding	ulceration	surgery radiotherapy	90%	
Stomach	possibly dietary factors occupational factors (inorganic dust – coal miners, pottery workers)	lymph nodes liver lung bone	loss of appetite weight loss	chronic indigestion anaemia vomiting blood in stools	surgery (radiotherapy, chemotherapy not usually effective)	7%	

Testis	may occur when testicle has failed to descend	lymph nodes lung abdomen	unusual swelling or pain in testicle	enlargement of testicle lump in testicle	surgery radiotherapy chemotherapy	85%
Womb (body of uterus)	oestrogen treatment at menopause	lung liver lymph nodes	bleeding after menopause	vaginal bleeding after intercourse abnormally heavy periods bleeding between periods	surgery radiotherapy	more than 50%

* in many cases there is no clear line to be drawn between early and advanced symptoms

‡ an individual's chances of survival may be quite different from the statistical 5-year survival rates, depending on many factors such as age at onset of cancer, stage of cancer at diagnosis, general health

ADVANCED CANCER

The goals of treatment for advanced cancers vary according to the extent of the cancer and with time. To begin with, the doctors may direct treatment towards giving the patient the longest remission possible, by bringing about, as far as can be detected, a total remission of the disease. If this succeeds, the patient should be able to live a normal life until, after an often unpredictable period of time, the disease returns.

In a number of kinds of cancer, treatment will produce a permanent remission in a small proportion of patients. If the disease does return, however, it is generally found to have become resistant to the remedies (hormones or cytotoxic drugs) used before. Other drugs and measures may be used to give the patient a further remission, but eventually the oncologist will find that he has no more shots left in his locker.

From then on, the treatment has a rather different goal: chiefly palliative, to minimise the symptoms, without attempting to clear away all evidence of the disease.

As the disease progresses, the treatment will become purely palliative. There are many symptom-relieving measures that can be used very effectively to enable the patient to feel reasonably comfortable.

Though patients with advanced cancer share common problems, it is extremely unlikely that any two people with incurable cancer will be treated in the same way, for these reasons:

○ Different tumours cause different disabilities: one kind may metastasise in the bones, so damaging the skeleton, another may be confined to the abdominal cavity, causing obstruction of the bowel or discomfort owing to excess of fluid. Moreover, people who have tumours of similar origin may experience quite different complications.

○ The treatment of these different manifestations depends on whether the cancer is slow- or fast-growing, whether it is responsive to drugs or to hormones, etc. The size and position of the tumour will determine whether localised treatment (surgery or radiation) will be used in addition to, or instead of, systemic drug or hormone therapy.

○ How long the doctors will carry on using curative measures must depend on the patient's own wishes and his readiness to undergo possibly distressing therapy. Before agreeing to such further therapy, a patient would be right to insist that the doctor gives some indication of what he is hoping to achieve, the chances of its being effective and the side-effects.

telling the bad news

There used to be a notion – now not so often met with – that people with advanced incurable cancer could and should be kept unaware of their condition. Their families would spend the last months bearing the burden of hiding the truth, in order to let the patient die in ignorance.

This notion originated in the days when there was no treatment, other than surgery, that was of any value. If a cancer was inoperable, that amounted to a death-sentence. The standard question from anyone told that they had inoperable cancer was: "How long have I got?" Nowadays more is generally known about cancer, and people are aware that a long remission or even cure is often possible.

There is now a new problem for families and doctors: telling someone who already knows he has cancer, that the disease has advanced past the point of curability. This may be because it was not observed early enough; or because treatment has failed to halt its progress; or because the tumour, thought to have been eliminated, has recurred or become widespread.

Telling the bad news may be more a matter of encouraging the sick person to ask the questions, giving openings which make asking easy and not shying away from them.

why the patient should be told the truth

When the patient's family and friends know the true state of affairs, keeping him in ignorance may create a barrier between them at a time when mutual support and comfort are most needed. The patient is likely to sense that he is the subject of a conspiracy of silence, and may become spiritually isolated from people who should be closest – physically isolated, too, if the burden of secrecy means that family and friends keep away.

For the same reason, a patient who knows the truth should be discouraged from 'sparing' the family by keeping them in ignorance: the feeling of having been deceived can only aggravate their grief.

Practical complications can arise from failing to tell someone that their time is short. There will be arrangements to make, to do with family, friends, work and finance. The prospect of dying can be eased to some extent by knowing that one's affairs are in order, and one's dependants provided for.

The sick person may also need to make mental and emotional provision. Religious people will want time to prepare themselves spiritually for death. Almost everyone will welcome a chance to adjust to the prospect, and to say their goodbyes; this applies equally to the survivors.

When the patient who has not been told becomes aware of the truth eventually, the bitterness of approaching death could be compounded by feeling that one has been cheated of the opportunity to make preparation.

Where the patient guesses the truth for himself, and asks the doctor outright for confirmation, he probably wants, and should receive, an honest answer. A sensitive doctor should be able to tell, from the tone of the question, whether such an answer is what is wanted, or – as sometimes happens – that the patient really wants to be comforted by vague assurances.

As for the patient's family, they will be better able to care for him if they can be warned about the likely progress of his physical decline and the probable symptoms, and if they are taught ways of relieving physical and mental anguish.

who should do the telling

There is no single answer: each situation must be thought out individually. At first glance, the doctor, especially the patient's own GP, may seem to be the most suitable person. The subject can be raised naturally by him, he is less emotionally involved, and he will have had some practice. But he may decide, from his knowledge of the circumstances, to tell close members of the family first, and decide with them whether he or they should do the telling. Or the best decision may be for the sufferer to hear the news first, so that he will not have cause to complain that he was the last to know.

People's reactions to being told that they have incurable cancer are bound to vary. Those who are looking after a cancer patient, and who know him best – his family, and his doctor – should consider how he is likely to take the news, whether with anxiety, depression, apathy or anger, and they should be prepared for any of these.

who should not be told

There are people who would prefer not to be told that their disease is incurable: it should be possible to gauge this from their response when the subject is cautiously broached and an opening is given which makes asking easy. The sufferer's need to protect himself by denial should then be respected, and the truth should not be forced on him. It may be that this need will change later, with the inevitable decline in his physical condition.

Some patients give unmistakable signals that they are content to have only a limited amount of information and explanation.

what the patient needs to know

In many cases, the patient's fear and anxiety is so overwhelming that, at the first telling, he cannot take in what he is being told. For this reason, many doctors prefer a close relative or a friend to be present. It may be a good idea to make a second appointment – the initial news is sometimes not taken in the first time.

On being told that their cancer is incurable, many people want to be told exactly what lies in store for them; how much life is left to them, and what its quality is likely to be. Advances in medicine make it possible for the doctor to assure them that even advanced cancers are to some extent treatable, if not curable, and to stress the positive aspect of what can be done.

No two explanations will be alike. Everyone has a store of notions, many of them ill-founded, about advanced cancer, picked up from the remembered experiences of friends or relations, from novels or magazines, from anecdotes, from television programmes. This means that everyone who can articulate his notions and fears will need a different explanation to set him straight.

What applies to one patient will not be true of another. For this reason, also, even though the doctor may have a fairly accurate idea of how long the sufferer is likely to survive, he is unlikely to give the patient a hard-and-fast prognosis. What may be more important for the patient is to know how endurable the rest of his life is likely to be after treatment – and also without further treatment.

Some patients may accept the information in a spirit of passivity close to apathy, others start by denying that what they are told can be true. Generally both change their attitude after a while, to a more active and positive one. When faced with the reality of the situation, they often resolve to defy the disease, and to accept any help and treatment that will allow them to live a relatively normal active life for as long as possible.

avoiding false cheer
Though the sick person should not be offered a firm date for the ending of his life, neither should the news of advanced cancer be accompanied by optimistic reassurance. Most advanced cancers eventually prove fatal: the sufferers are going to die, perhaps not very soon, yet much sooner than they once supposed. It is cruel to delude them with hopeful predictions, which will have to be withdrawn as the months go by.

Instead, the sufferer should be helped to readjust his expectations. Psychotherapeutic counselling can be useful in encouraging him to use his own resources in coping with the disease, whether it is a question of enduring unpleasant treatments, or of dealing with social and personal problems, or of accepting a gradual decline in health. Group therapy can help cancer sufferers to share their anxieties, discuss things they have not talked about to their family or to doctors.

The patient will have to learn to substitute realistic short-term aims for long-term plans. These aims could be anything from finishing a piece of work, to living long enough to reach an important anniversary or to attend a family celebration. The satisfaction of achieving these can do much to improve the quality of the sufferer's remaining life.

terminal cancer

By the time it has become clear that the disease can no longer be held in check, the patient may have learnt to accept the inevitability of death. There may still be periods of panic, despair and feeling isolated, and the patient's family, friends and doctor should do all they can to support him through these bad times.

dealing with the physical problems

This is an area in which a great deal can be done by doctors and nurses to make patients feel more comfortable.

the relief of pain
Though pain is the first problem one thinks of in connection with cancer, a considerable proportion of people with advanced cancer suffer no pain, even when close to death, and some feel pain only intermittently.

The doctor's first task will be to identify the source of the pain and to assess its type and intensity. If it is localised, the appropriate treatment may be radiotherapy; if it is more general, cytotoxic drugs or hormones may be used. All these treatments work by temporarily controlling the growth of cancer cells.

There are many drugs, that are used simply to control pain; they range in strength from the familiar analgesics, aspirin and paracetamol, through codeine, to powerful narcotic painkillers based on morphine or diamorphine (heroin). The choice depends in the first instance on the doctor's experience and his assessment of the patient's needs, how effective the drug proves, and how acceptable to the patient. Most analgesics taken over a long period of time tend to cause constipation, and some cause nausea or sleepiness. A drug that helps some patients may cause intolerable side-effects in others.

Morphine and diamorphine are only two of the narcotic painkillers. The problem with some of these is that they are addictive (which is largely irrelevant for a terminally ill patient) and that the dose needs to be continually increased to maintain effectiveness. However, even this problem can be got round, as most doctors who care for terminally ill patients have now acquired great expertise in administering pain-reducing drugs.

If patients cared for at home or in hospital are not getting adequate pain or symptom relief, they or the relatives should ask to see a specialist (for example a specialist in pain relief). Some patients, especially at home, suffer avoidable pain, or are drugged more than they need to be, because their GP is not knowledgeable about this. The problem may not just be the drug: the frequency with which it is given makes a difference.

It has been observed that patients who are promised adequate analgesia, with plenty of morphia if necessary, eventually feel so reassured that they come to suffer less pain, and so their requirement for these drugs does not necessarily increase.

constipation
This can be caused by the action of the tumour on the abdominal cavity, an inadequate diet from loss of appetite, or be the result of radiotherapy, chemotherapy, or the analgesics themselves. Constipation can be relieved by laxatives taken by mouth, or

occasionally by suppositories or enemas. For a person who is being cared for at home, the GP can arrange for the district nurse (community nurse) to come and administer these.

loss of appetite, weakness and lethargy

This is a major problem in many, though not all, cases of advanced cancer: patients refuse food at a time when they most need to keep up their strength. Nobody has yet succeeded in finding out exactly why this happens, but it is chiefly responsible for terminal patients' characteristic loss of weight. Problems such as difficulty in swallowing should be discussed with the dietitian (and the doctor). Dietitians employed by hospitals can give valuable advice on providing the sick person with a diet which is both appetising and nourishing. The aim is to get the patient to eat a good balance of protein, carbohydrates and fats, adding up to enough calories to prevent weight loss. Plenty of fibre (fruit and vegetables) in the diet may help to prevent constipation.

Not eating enough may be one of the causes of weakness and lethargy. These symptoms may be mild at first, but can gradually increase to the point where they hamper the patient's normal activities. Attention to diet can help. Doctors sometimes pre-scribe appetite stimulants such as steroid hormones – in small doses to avoid the side-effects of putting on fat, fluid retention or wasting of bone and muscle.

other symptoms

Some symptoms are associated with particular types of cancer. For instance, anaemia arising from bone marrow damage can result in shortness of breath, and so can damage to the lungs caused by a tumour.

Often a lung does not function properly because fluid has collected in the pleural cavity around the lungs, pressing on them so that they cannot expand: this too causes shortness of breath. The condition is usually easy to relieve, either by drugs or by drawing out the fluid (aspiration) through a hollow needle inserted through the chest wall; this is done under local anaesthetic and causes only mild discomfort. A similar procedure is used in the case of build-up of fluid in the abdomen.

reporting symptoms
It is important for patients with advanced cancer (as indeed for people with early cancer) to report any new symptoms, especially if they are in remission. Some symptoms may be frightening but have trivial causes; on the other hand, minor symptoms may indicate serious complications, such as the ending of remission, and so the patient should lose no time in telling the doctor about them.

psychological problems

The chief ones are depression and anxiety. They can often be relieved by psychotherapy or counselliing. This generally requires 'one-to-one' contact between therapist and patient. It may be possible to arrange this privately for the patient at home.

In a hospital, patients are cared for by teams of doctors chiefly concerned with physical aspects of the disease. But even there, individual counselling or psychotherapy can be arranged for specific problems. Anti-depressant drugs may also be very effective.

It is important for the doctors to be aware that the patient is depressed. Since they are not familiar with his everyday moods, this may escape their notice, and it may be up to the patient's family to be the first to notice and to alert them. Signs of depression include lack of energy, loss of interest, disturbed sleep – adding up to an overall change of mood.

self-help and support groups
Counselling is not giving advice; it is helping people to put into words their fears and anxieties and to adjust to them. Counselling may also be on a group basis. There exist various organisations, mostly voluntary, whose purpose is to help people with cancer (whether it is curable or incurable), and also sometimes

their families, to come to terms with what has befallen them. They can also help them to cope with some of the personal and social problems that accompany the disease. Amongst the worst of these is a feeling of isolation because of friends who no longer act naturally and seem embarrassed or stay away.

Some drugs used in treating cancer cause loss of libido, and depression in itself can be the cause of loss of interest in one's sex life. Probably this happens more often than anyone knows, because patients are reluctant to talk about this delicate subject, and so are their partners – the doctors may not think of raising it, unless prompted. Treatment of the depression by whatever means may greatly improve matters.

In late illness, the decline in the patient's general health is likely to be the cause of loss of sexual function. It should, however, be possible, and may be comforting, to have physical closeness.

terminal care – at home, or in hospital?

Both of these have their advantages and their drawbacks when it comes to caring for dying cancer patients.

Many different specialists take part in caring for cancer patients: doctors, specialist cancer nurses, occupational therapists, physiotherapists, dietitians, etc. When the patient is being cared for at home, the activities of all of these are co-ordinated by the GP. Specialist care is, however, easier to arrange when the patient is in hospital, which has the equipment and facilities for the various treatments available on the spot.

But the patient in hospital, being cared for by teams of medical and paramedical staff, often feels that he cannot regard any of the doctors as being individually concerned with him, and that none of them has much time for building up a closer contact. Individual, loving care is more likely to be found at home.

But members of one's own family, however willing and eager, are not expert, and may well be strained beyond their strength, both in body and in mind, by looking after someone they love who is dying. Unlike doctors and nurses, they are not accustomed to such work, and cannot assume an impersonal attitude. In any case, many patients do not have friends and relations able and willing to shoulder the burden.

the hospice: what it is and what it does

The hospice movement was started in Britain about 20 years ago, for the express purpose of caring for the incurably ill and dying, and also of helping their families through the last months or weeks, and their time of bereavement.

The care can be given in the hospice itself, or in the patient's own home: teams of cancer nurses (such as the Macmillan nurses' home care team) provide the link between the hospice, the home and the GP.

Admission to a hospice is generally made through the patient's own doctor and there is no financial barrier to the admission of those in need of care.

Hospices, though they may be religious foundations, accept people of every variety of belief, or none. They care for people suffering from any disease, not just cancer, for whom nothing more can be done in the way of a cure. The aim of the hospice doctors and nurses is to relieve pain and other symptoms of bodily dissolution so that patients and their families can make the most of the time they have left to spend together.

Analgesics and other drugs are used in carefully calculated doses to deaden pain without stupefying the sick person, and this treatment is continuous, so that there are no spells of returning pain to be dreaded. The other symptoms, such as constipation, shortness of breath, etc, are also controlled. The patients and their families are offered counselling, secular and also religious, as needed: patients are helped to face death with some serenity and an unclouded mind, recognisably the same person the family has always known. Life support machinery is not offered, so that no one needs to dread being kept alive artificially.

incurable cancer and the quality of life

Life is not a matter of not being dead: many elements, physiological, psychological, social and spiritual contribute to make up the intangible factor called 'the quality of life'. It defies evaluation, and is different for each person. Life on any terms is not what many, perhaps most, people would settle for.

ALTERNATIVE AND COMPLEMENTARY THERAPIES

'Alternative' is the name given to remedies and treatments for disease that are not included in conventional medical practice, or that have not undergone the rigorous controlled tests, both laboratory and clinical, which are required for conventional drugs and treatments. They are referred to as 'complementary' when they are intended to reinforce, not replace, conventional therapy.

Many practitioners of complementary medicine feel that there is no 'alternative' system. What is seen as 'alternative' should be recognised for what it is – a remedying of the gaps in orthodox medicine and extension of treatment into areas and levels of existence which orthodox medicine does not reach at present. They assert that what is needed if cancer is ever to be overcome is a team effort by conventional and orthodox therapists working together in harmony with those now labelled alternative/complementary, both in prevention and in treatment.

The range of unconventional treatments is wide, and includes dietary regimes; herbal or 'natural' pharmacological remedies; vitamin therapy; acupuncture; hypnotherapy; meditation and other mental disciplines, spiritual healing. Holistic medicine, which aims to treat not just the disease but the whole body and mind together, includes elements of several of these treatments.

Cancer, perhaps more than any other disease, has given rise to a proliferating range of unconventional treatments. There are numerous reasons for this, such as

○ modern conventional cancer treatments are passive, that is, patients have things done to them and so welcome treatment in which they themselves are encouraged to take active measures

○ there is feeling of disappointment that modern medicine has failed to come up with a cure for cancer, which would be as easy to take and as reliable in its effects as antibiotics have been in the case of infectious diseases

○ for many cancers modern therapies have not significantly improved the survival rate (a fact particularly stressed by supporters of alternative treatments)

○ the notion exists that modern medicine is on the wrong track, having a blinkered approach to cancer, and that the more imaginative approach of alternative therapists is more likely to succeed

○ the unpleasant and sometimes mutilating nature of some cancer treatments, may make the extension of life they give seem hardly worth the misery involved

○ many people believe that there is a cure in nature for every disease, and that remedies that are 'natural' in the sense of being derived from things that grow, are more likely to offer a cure than laboratory-engineered drugs, or 'unnatural' interference with the body through surgery or radiation.

why orthodox medicine is hostile

Modern medicine now thinks in terms not of 'a cure for cancer', but of as many ways of successfully treating cancer as there are types of cancer. The notion that conventional medicine has failed to eliminate cancer ignores the fact that some cancers which used to be almost invariably fatal (such as acute lymphatic leukaemia and Hodgkin's disease in children and young adults) are now almost routinely successfully treated (the 5-year survival rates for Hodgkin's disease has risen from 39% in the 1950's to 80% in the 1970's; for acute lymphatic leukaemia the improvement in that period has been from 4% to 50%).

In many cases, alternative treatments are sought as treatments of last resort: people who have been told that their disease is not treatable are most likely to be ready to try some other therapy, however bizarre, out of a feeling that they have nothing to lose. It would be heartless to criticise such a decision. However, a number of people resort to alternative medicine in early disease, because they are suspicious of orthodox medicine, and impressed by the claims of alternative therapists. It is cases like this that most provoke the hostility of orthodox therapists, especially if the cancer is of a type with a proven track record of successful treatments. If the alternative treatment disappoints, the patient's cancer will have had time to grow and proliferate, and become more difficult to treat by conventional methods.

One problem with unorthodox therapy is the absence of rigorous proof of its effectiveness. Most of the treatments available have not undergone the sort of trials that are demanded of orthodox remedies. The few that have been so tested have performed disappointingly in the trials (but it has been claimed that these trials were not fairly conducted).

A notable characteristic of some advocates of alternative treatments is lack of objectivity. There is a considerable body of literature promoting this or that treatment, and giving, in each case, numerous case histories of success. What these books do not usually dwell on, however, is the failures, and so they tend to give the impression that the treatment in question works in almost every case. Not even the most effective orthodox treatments are expected to succeed with every patient, only a statistically significant proportion. Records of clinical trials list failures as well as successes, while unorthodox healers tend to be reticent on the subject of the former. When failure is admitted, it tends to be blamed on the fact that the patient started the treatment too late, having been waylaid by the claims of orthodox medicine, which had destroyed his natural powers of recovery.

Where there is an apparent cure, there is the question of whether it is the result of the alternative treatment, and whether it is permanent. Some improvement may be due to the working of the 'placebo effect': the very fact of being treated may have a beneficial effect, but this psychologically induced improvement is not usually lasting.

Moreover, it is a feature of cancer that spontaneous remissions do (very rarely) occur, and sometimes last for several years. It is difficult to be sure whether any improvement was actually due to the treatment.

alternative therapy as a way of life

Many alternative treatments require the patient to adopt a new mode of living, which may involve not only a particular diet, but a new system of exercise and even of thinking. The idea behind this is that disease is the loss of a natural equilibrium in the patient, caused by living in a harmful way, and that the new way of life will redress the balance, and so banish the disease. Mental resistance to the disease is taught as a reinforcement to the physical regime.

In this way, the responsibility for the cure is laid on the patient, a notion that many people understandably welcome: in the hands of orthodox doctors, with their battery of highly technical treatments, many people feel helpless and passive, and would prefer to feel that they are able to help themselves. The drawbacks of this approach is that the alternative life-styles are often quite demanding. Everyone who tries them is likely now and again to fail to meet these demands. If the treatment fails, the patient may feel that he has failed himself, so adding the burden of guilt to that of failing health.

The alternative mental and physical regimes are usually recommended for prevention, as well as cure: if everyone lived rightly from their earlier days, there would be no disease. This philosophy should not be dismissed out of hand: there is epidemiological evidence to show that many cancers are connected with the way some people eat, work and live (smoking is a case in point) and it is likely that future research will confirm that many cancers are induced by people's life-styles, and therefore can be prevented by changing these.

vitamin therapy

The claims that a large intake of some vitamins can prevent cancer have already been discussed. The same vitamins are also often claimed to have a curative effect on established cancer.

vitamin A

There is no evidence acceptable to most orthodox doctors that carotene from which the body manufactures retinol (vitamin A) or the vitamin itself, taken in amounts larger than found in a normal diet, will have any effect on malignant disease. Taking large doses of retinol in pill form can cause liver damage, the warning signs are yellowing skin and headache.

Beta-carotene, in the form of carrot juice or as capsules, as recommended by many alternative therapy systems, is non-toxic, however; at worst it will turn the skin yellow temporarily.

vitamin E

This vitamin has been shown to inhibit the transformation of nitrites and nitrates in food into carcinogenic nitrosamines, but it has not been found to have any effect on tumours induced by nitrosamines, in laboratory animals. Failing further evidence, no verdict can be definitely given on its effectiveness, but additional vitamin E is not advisable in cases of breast and other hormone-dependent cancers.

vitamin C

The highest claims have been made for this vitamin, notably by Dr Linus Pauling, a Nobel laureate in chemistry (who has also advocated vitamin C as therapy for the common cold, a treatment which many people swear by). Vitamin C, in huge doses (as much as 35 grams a day) is said to have been found effective in arresting the growth of tumours in human patients, and in causing the tumours to regress, even, in some cases, when they were advanced and had metastasised.

In 1984 the National Cancer Institute in the USA carried out controlled trials of vitamin C, which failed to demonstrate its effectiveness. These trials have been criticised, however, on methodological grounds, and it may be that the last word on this subject has not yet been said.

Linus Pauling and his collaborator Dr Ewan Cameron suggest, moreover, that vitamin C is a useful adjunct to chemotherapy and radiotherapy, reducing side-effects and speeding the healing of normal tissues. Since vitamin C is tolerated by the body even in large doses, there seems to be no reason why anyone under going conventional cancer therapy should not try this out for himself.

laetrile (amygdalin, or nitriloside)

This is also called vitamin B17 but is not actually a vitamin. It is made from the kernels of apricot stones or from bitter almonds, and contains quite a lot of cyanide, together with a substance given the name of benzaldehyde. Advocates of laetrile claim that its cancer-destroying action is released by contact with an enzyme produced by cancer cells and that normal cells are protected from this effect by another enzyme.

In clinical trials carried out on laetrile in the USA, no evidence was found of any effect on cancer tumours. There is some doubt about the methodology of these trials, too, and also of whether the laetrile used was biologically active. Laetrile has been claimed to be non-toxic, but in fact its cyanide content makes it quite toxic in large doses. It has not been licensed for use in the USA or in this country. Even its advocates say that for laetrile to be therapeutically effective, it would have to be administered by injection, since oral doses of the requisite size would be very toxic.

selenium

This element has, like vitamin E, a role to play in controlling the effects of oxygen in the tissues, but there is no evidence that it is effective in treating cancer. It is toxic if taken in amounts much larger than the trace amounts found in the normal diet.

dietary therapy

Various systems exist of treating cancer by means of diet. They are mostly founded on the same concept, namely that of bolster-ing the body's own healing powers. Cancer is said to occur when the body's own immune defences fail. Carcinogens in the envi-ronment are constantly invading the organism, but in a healthy body which has been properly nourished, the immune system is able to meet this challenge, identifying cancer cells as 'non-self' as soon as they appear, and destroying them; in an unhealthy body, the immune system fails to rise to the challenge, and opens the gates to cancer and other diseases. The diets recommended are claimed to work by restoring the body's natural defences, which can then turn against any malignant tumours and hold back their growth, or destroy them completely.

In support of this theory, it is pointed out that in a group of people exposed to the same carcinogen levels, some are unaffected. Not all heavy smokers get lung cancer, and industrial diseases do not attack every single worker in an industry. The reason why some escape could be the superior efficiency of their immune system.

Dietary therapies have many features in common. They describe the eating of:

○ large amounts of fresh, preferably raw, vegetables and fruit; if possible, organically grown without artificial fertilisers and pesticides
○ little or no fat in any form
○ little or no meat
○ no salt or sugar
○ no coffee or tea.

Pauling and Cameron suggest that dietary therapies of this kind owe their successes to the large amounts of vitamin C which they provide in the fruit and vegetables.

Those regimes which are not wholly vegetarian or even vegan (excluding all animal products, such as eggs, milk or honey), usually ban red meat in favour of modest amounts of fish and poultry, which are lower in fat. Eggs, which contain a good deal of fat, are not recommended.

Some regimes exclude cereal products, others allow them if organically grown and unprocessed (brown rice, wholemeal bread, etc). Wine and spirits are either banned or greatly restricted.

the Gerson therapy
This system was pioneered by the late Dr Max Gerson on the basis of clinical experience in Germany and the USA, for the prevention and cure of cancer. It is at present undergoing clinical trials in Austria. It claims to destroy tumours by restoring the efficiency of the immune system and the liver, and restoring the depleted levels of potassium within the cells, due at least in part to overconsumption of salt. As the cancer is destroyed, the body is detoxified by the removal from the blood-stream, especially through stimulation of bile secretion, of the toxic waste products so produced.

The diet consists chiefly of fruit and vegetables – eaten steamed, raw, or in the form of juice. Potassium supplements are taken, also liver extract, or liquefied raw liver, mixed with carrot juice. No salt or fats are allowed. Caffeine enemas are administered for detoxification, but coffee or tea may not be drunk. It is emphasised that the therapy must be taken as a whole, not piecemeal. It is quite demanding of time and effort, and special appliances, not the standard blenders, must be used for preparation.

the Pritikin diet
This was developed primarily for the prevention and cure of coronary heart disease, but has now begun to be recommended as beneficial in cancer. It is a low-fat regime, which stresses wholegrain cereals and pulses, fruit and vegetables, and discourages processed foods. It forbids eggs, sugar and salt; fish, lean meat and poultry are allowed in restricted amounts.

macrobiotic diet
This is an even more limited diet, depending largely on wholegrain cereals such as whole wheat, brown rice, barley, etc. Some, but not all vegetables are included; among those which are excluded are potatoes, tomatoes, aubergines, courgettes and spinach. Some (not all) pulses are allowed, and sea-vegetables, chiefly of Japanese origin (for example kombu, wakame) are

positively recommended. Tropical fruit, such as mangoes and bananas, is forbidden, while locally grown fresh fruit is allowed in small amounts. The only animal protein allowed must come from white fish, and is severely restricted. No eggs; no dairy produce; no sugar; seasalt only. Water, preferably spring water, not iced, is the only drink.

In addition to dietary rules, there are a good many others, such as not watching colour television (because of radiation), not cooking with electricity, and substituting rub-downs with hot towels for having baths or showers.

holistic medicine

This takes its name from the Greek: *holos* – whole, and is the form for therapies (for all diseases, not only cancer) that are directed towards the patient's mind as well as his body (the whole body, not just the diseased part), regarding them as an indivisible whole. Orthodox medicine acknowledges, to some extent, an interplay between mind and body in causing disease, and the label 'psychosomatic' (greek: *psyche* – soul, *soma* – body) has been coined for diseases in which this occurs. In practice, it is the physical side of illness that tends to receive most attention, even when it is an illness like asthma, known to be connected with emotional states.

This is not invariably so: an increasing number of orthodox physicians now favour the holistic approach, but it is the advocates of holistic therapies who most insist on the unity of mind and body. They recommend meditation and other mental disciplines as having a role to play in combating disease equal to that of the recommended dietary regimes and physical treatments.

The rationale of this is that stressful events in people's lives can be as damaging as exposure to harmful substances in breaking down the body's defences and allowing disease to take hold. The most devastating stress factor is considered to be the death of a spouse. Tests carried out in the USA show that a spouse's death usually reduces the efficiency of the survivor's immune system for some months, sometimes beyond recovery. Other life-disturbing events, such as the death of a parent or a child, loss of job, moving house, are said to have a similar effect to a lesser degree.

Studies are being carried out in Britain and in other countries in Europe to find out more about a possible link between personal misfortunes, such as divorce or widowhood, and the onset of breast cancer.

If states of mind have the power to depress the body's defences, they may also be able to build them up again. Studies have shown that survival rates in breast cancer are highest in women who tackle the disease in a fighting spirit, and lowest in passive women, who are unable to express feelings of anger, sorrow or resentment. The question arises whether someone with a passive personality can be helped to become more positively-minded. Holistic therapists believe that this is possible and that attitudes of hopelessness and despair can be changed to hope and confidence.

In the world of orthodox medicine, the precise relationship between the cancer and the patient's state of mind is a matter of controversy, but most doctors (holistic or conventional) would agree that patients are strongly to be encouraged to adopt positive attitudes. Holistic therapists design their treatments on this principle.

Although there are differences in details, and sometimes in emphasis, the main factors of holistic medicine are: diet and dietary supplements; physical treatment, mental and spiritual therapy. All are intended to work towards the same goal: the strengthening of the immune system, to enable it to recognise, attack and destroy the tumour cells.

the dietary regime

This is nutritional support of the immune system by diet; this must be practical and accessible and not allowed to become a further source of stress. Vegetables and fruit, organically grown and freshly picked, are the basis of the diet: eaten raw or lightly cooked, and never tinned, or preserved. The diet includes wholegrain cereals, pulses, seeds (whole or sprouted) and nuts. Small amounts of chicken and fish are allowed, though not in the earliest stages of therapy – it may be necessary to be vegetarian for the first 6 to 8 weeks. Dairy foods are sometimes allowed, if low in fat. Salt, sugar, chocolate, coffee (even decaffeinated) are forbidden, sometimes also tea. Tap water should be replaced by bottled spring water.

Fibre is recommended, to speed the transit time of food residue through the bowel, to keep any toxins in it from prolonged contact with the bowel wall.

dietary supplements

All holistic therapies recommend vitamin and mineral supplements. Some stress certain vitamins more than others, but there is general agreement on the value of vitamin A, given as carrot juice or as retinol in amounts below toxic levels. Vitamin C is also given in mega-doses. Supplements may be given of any or all of the B vitamins, vitamins D and E, zinc, potassium, selenium, lithium, iodine, calcium, magnesium. Laetrile is sometimes given.

physical treatment

This includes elimination of as much of the cancerous material as possible, preferably by surgery. Radiation or chemotherapy may be employed at a level low enough not to destroy the immune system.

Some holistic therapists believe that the BCG (*bacille Calmette-Guérin*) vaccine, used to prevent tuberculosis by stimulating antibody reaction, is also valuable in bolstering the immune system against cancer cells. (This is also used by some orthodox practitioners in the treatment of leukaemia and malignant melanoma.) Some also consider the administration of enzymes an important aspect of holistic therapy, given by mouth or by retention enema or directly injected into the tumour site.

mental and spiritual therapy

This rests on the belief that some event (or events) in the patient's life, past or present, has been the cause of trauma or injury to his mental and emotional state or to the person's perception of or reaction to the event(s), and has depressed his vital forces. As a result, he has subconsciously lost most or all of his will to live and conspired against himself to open the gates to disease. The aim of therapy is to detect and heal this trauma, restoring the desire to go on living, which will be reflected in the patient's improving physical condition. Among the methods used are:

psychotherapy, both individual and in groups, to identify crisis points in the patient's life from earliest childhood onwards, and to help him find a resolution

counselling, to help the person explore his own feelings, to counter negative and despairing attitudes, and replace them by a positive, optimistic, determined outlook

deep relaxation and meditation (singly or in groups): the technique, which has to be learned, is intended to restore peace of mind. Patients are taught how to control and discipline the mind so that anxious fearful thoughts are not allowed to dominate; then positive thoughts can be marshalled, and the patient comes to feel that he is in control of his body and its reactions. This is related to:

biofeedback, a technique taught by some therapists, which encourages the patient to achieve control of his mind by monitoring his level of relaxation; physical processes usually thought to be involuntary, such as blood pressure and heartbeat, may also be controlled

auto-hypnosis, a technique in which the patient learns to turn the power of suggestion upon his own body, commanding it to reject and destroy the tumour

visualisation, a form of auto-hypnosis in which the patient is taught to visualise his tumour, and to concentrate on an image of it being attacked and demolished or melting away and disappearing.

The advocates of holistic therapy vary in the emphasis they lay on the mental aspect of it; some see it as simply an adjunct to healing, while others represent it as a spiritually transforming experience, akin to religious conversion.

other kinds of complementary therapy

Some therapies are used as reinforcements to holistic therapies, but may also be used as complete treatments in themselves.

hypnotherapy is the treatment of disease by the power of suggestion, applied to a patient in a trance state. It is used by many orthodox practitioners in the treatment of asthma and other diseases, and as a help in alleviating pain.

acupuncture, deriving from Chinese medical practice, is the treatment of diseases by the insertion of fine needles at various points of the body, which are said to be points along energy channels, in order to promote changes in the pattern of energy flow, and so to affect the condition of other parts of the body.

healing and spiritual healing

There is no accounting for the gift of healing: it appears to be inborn, like absolute pitch, and not even those who have it understand exactly how it works. They usually explain it in terms of a force or energy, of unknown, perhaps divine origin: a healing power, of which they are the conduit, and which they can transmit to others by their touch; or sometimes even without touching or even being in the same place as the patient. The latter is called 'absent healing'.

The term 'spiritual' is used here for those healers who claim that their powers come from God: some have a specific religious affiliation, while others are inter-denominational. The term 'healers' is used for those who are somewhat agnostic about the source of their gift, and demand no religious faith from their patients. These patients are not expected to remain passive: they must take an active part in the process by willing themselves to get well, and willing their disease to disappear. Thus meditation and visualisation may be involved in the healing process, for the relief of stress, and to involve the patient in his own recovery.

It has been found that it is only the highly motivated who stay the course of treatment on these terms. This bears out other unorthodox therapists' belief that getting well is to some extent a question of genuinely wanting to get well.

the case for and against alternative and complementary medicine

The practitioners of unconventional therapies have tended to be dismissed, in the past (and still are, in many quarters) as either charlatans, cynically cheating the gullible sick with quack remedies, or fantasists, attributing quasi-magical powers to useless regimens, and claiming credit for spontaneous remissions. Orthodox therapists assert that those ill with cancer are particularly vulnerable to false claims, being in a condition to clutch at anything that offers hope; and that this may lead them to abandon conventional treatments which have a good chance of success, for illusory ones. They point out that alternative treatments do not undergo the sort of trials by which the value of orthodox therapies is judged, and that where trials have been done, no efficacy was discovered.

Unconventional therapists counter this by claiming that their treatments have never been fairly tested; they claim that the orthodox controlled trial is inappropriate. Such tests as have been done were carried out by people whose whole careers were linked to the use of technologically-developed, costly cytotoxic drugs, and who thus had a vested interest in the failure of other treatments. They further say that the tests were done on people with advanced cancer who had already received radiotherapy and chemotherapy, treatments which reduce the ability of the immune system to repel invaders, and that their own treatments cannot wholly restore this, even though they can often alleviate the symptoms and prolong life in an acceptable way.

Many unorthodox therapists would like wholly to replace the

term 'alternative' by 'complementary', asserting that they want to work alongside orthodox treatments, not to replace them. They are generally agreed as to the value of surgery in removing considerable areas of tumour tissue, provided that it is not too mutilating.

Holistic practitioners' main criticism is of the damage done by cytotoxic drugs, which affect every cell in the body including the sites of origin of the white blood cells. Where the chance of a cure by this means is poor, it is felt to be wrong to provoke distressing side-effects.

It is hard to reconcile the two approaches completely and to consider as complementary the holistic approach which holds that cytotoxic drugs do more harm than good and the orthodox approach which relies heavily on the efficacy of cytotoxic drugs.

gentle ways

Alternative therapists are probably on strongest ground when they point to the gentleness of their methods. The dietary regimes, whether for prevention or for cure, chime with orthodox medical recommendations for a healthy diet: low in fat, high in fibre, lacking no vitamins. Nor is it easy to see how relaxation, meditation, and psychotherapy, especially group therapy in the company of fellow-sufferers, can do anything but good. In fact, they very often seem to do good, if not always in curing, then in prolonging and enhancing the quality of life or helping patients to come to terms with the prospect of death. Alternative therapy is said to ease the discomforts of conventional therapy, and enable the incurable patient to make the most of his remaining time, and die with dignity. On the whole, there seems little reason why its methods should not be followed even in early cancer, and certainly in advanced disease, as an addition to the orthodox medical armoury.

not so gentle

It is true that the demands of some alternative treatments may be found too taxing by many. For instance, the Gerson treatment is generally agreed to require constant nursing attention and special equipment (and can probably only be carried out in a Gerson-style clinic). There may be other inconveniences: some people could feel that doing without tea or coffee reduces the quality of life they are trying to maintain. Some therapists have touched the verge of dottiness by forbidding the use of deodorants and detergents, and demanding that television should be watched in a mirror, the set being shielded with bricks, to avoid radiation.

patient helps himself

Holistic therapists stress the role played by the patient in his recovery, and insist that nothing less than a wholehearted commitment on his part will do. This could be a valuable counter to the feeling of helplessness that many people feel when caught up in high-technology therapy. But it is the therapist's duty not to make the patient feel guilty if the treatment fails, let alone feel that he is dying through his own fault.

Many orthodox medical people think that the alternative practitioners place too much faith in the body's immune system counteracting disease. Some holistic therapy claims that the patient's immune status can be improved to an extent that he will now be able to reject his tumour by some immunological mechanism. This is where the evidence is absent at the moment. Active immunotherapy has yet to be a proven method of cancer treatment. There is considerable interest in the scientific community in new approaches to immunology. Money is being spent on these approaches but, sadly, they have yet to show results which are in any way comparable with the older methods of surgery, radiotherapy and chemotherapy. It would be misleading to suggest that immunotherapy is a real alternative to those older methods. That is not to say that it may not have some complementary role.

more research

The Research Council for Complementary Medicine, many of whose members have the highest medical qualifications, is embarking on a series of research projects to put to the test the claims of some forms of unorthodox healing, with respect to some diseases. Cancer is not, at present, included, except in relation to spiritual healing, but it may, perhaps, be considered in later projects. One eventual result could be the putting of unorthodox therapists on a properly professional footing, with qualifications recognised by orthodox medicine.

medical homeopathy

The treatment of disease by homeopathic methods has affinities with both conventional and unconventional medicine. The principles and methods of homeopathy were first propounded towards the end of the 18th century, and for many years were regarded with suspicion by orthodox medicine. However, there has been a gradual change of attitude. Homeopathy has now achieved official recognition. In 1956 the Faculty of Homeopathy was founded by Act of Parliament to offer training (2 years) in homeopathic principles and methods to doctors already qualified in orthodox medicine. The letters MF(Hom) – Member of the Faculty of Homeopathy – indicate that a doctor has received such training.

There is a register of homeopathic medical practitioners. Some offer conventional as well as homeopathic treatment under the National Health Service.

However, the unconventional side of this system of therapy lies in the fact that one does not have to be a doctor to become a homeopathic practitioner. There is a second category of training available to lay people (though these often have some other sort of medical or paramedical qualification, such as nursing, or osteopathy). This training is also officially recognised; it lasts four years, and the practitioners are also registered.

Medical homeopaths do not recommend, however, that lay practitioners who are not qualified to use specialised diagnostic techniques, such as blood testing, should undertake the treatment of diseases such as cancer.

Homeopathy (from the Greek, *homoios*: similar) is the treatment of disease on the principle of 'like cures like'. Symptoms are treated with minute amounts of substances which, in larger amounts, would produce the same symptoms. When the patient's symptom matches that produced by a drug, herb or other substance, that drug or substance is said to be homeopathic to the disease. It is administered in a highly diluted form; paradoxically, this is called 'potentisation', because the effectiveness of the remedy is said to increase with the degree of dilution. The minute doses are claimed to be so effective because of being highly specific in their action, unlike the orthodox cytotoxic drugs, and other conventional remedies.

X-ray therapy has been adopted as part of the homeopathic treatment of cancer. X-rays are considered to be homeopathic to cancer, because they can induce it, and are therefore used – in low doses – in treating it.

Some homeopathic doctors, particularly in Switzerland, use Iscador, a 'potentised' preparation of mistletoe, in treating cancer. It is reputed to retard the growth of the cancer cells, and to increase the local tissue resistance to their spread. It is admitted to be toxic, but much less so than the orthodox cytotoxic drugs, and should only be prescribed by medical homeopaths.

Homeopathic practitioners understand the term 'symptoms' in a very wide sense. Everything about the patient, including personality, temperament, outlook, past experience, even physical appearance, is taken into consideration in diagnosing and prescribing, so that two patients with apparently identical conditions may be prescribed quite different remedies. Homeopathic practitioners assert that they treat the patient and not the disease: the building up of a complete picture of the patient is the most important part of treatment. So homeopathy is also a holistic therapy.

THE OUTLOOK FOR CANCER

Everyone must be aware that there is such a thing as cancer research, and that it is heavily dependent on charity: if only because of the proliferation of fund-raising charity shops, or the collecting tins thrust under their noses. And anyone who reads newspapers or watches television, knows that cancer is news.

When someone announces some small advance in therapy, this is usually hailed as a breakthrough, however untried and unconfirmed. Eventually one comes to scan the miracle cure of the month with a degree of cynicism – unless one is a sufferer, that is: each successive 'breakthrough' sees the switchboard of the hospital concerned jammed with calls from cancer victims or their relations, pleading to be included in the clinical trials.

what exactly is being researched?

Basically, the investigation of cancer has two aims: finding the cause (or causes) of cancer, and finding a cure (or cures). Obviously, the two fields of research are related: if more were known about the origin, nature and behaviour of cancer cells, science would find it that much easier to devise ways of preventing cancer, and of stemming and reversing the uncontrolled growth of tumour cells. But such fundamental research is a long-term business, which may not show results for many years, and cancer patients need immediate help. So a good deal of research is devoted to looking for new remedies.

Advances may be refinements of existing treatments, for instance, new versions of cytotoxic drugs, which are just as effective as the old ones, without causing patients the same distress. Or they may be new treatments altogether, like the much-heralded Interleukin-2. Or known drugs may be made more effective with the help of monoclonal antibodies, for example. Such research shows results on a comparatively short time scale, but the step from the laboratory to treatment and the clinic takes time. (New drugs and remedies have to be tested for effectiveness and safety - that is also why new miracle remedies may be discarded when it is found that they do not live up to their promise.)

research into the nature of cancer

This is now mostly concentrated in the field of molecular biology. Each cell of the human body carries a set of instructions for growing and reproducing, encoded in its cellular DNA, the material of inheritance; it is therefore hoped that by the study of genes, which are units of DNA, it can be found out what sort of flaw causes cells to proliferate out of control.

It is possible that the cells are receiving garbled instructions. This concept is developed in the study of growth factors, chemical substances which unite with protein receptors on the surfaces of cells, signalling to them to start and also to stop multiplying. (This growth factor mechanism operates in the case of wounds and other injuries, when new cells are needed to replace destroyed ones.) It is postulated that viruses can pervert the growth factor signals, causing the genes which act as the cells' switchgear to become oncogenes: that is, genes which cause cancer by failing to switch off the multiplication process. It appears that when certain viruses invade cells, they can pick up some of the cells' genetic material: they can transfer this to cells elsewhere in the body, so causing them to receive the wrong instructions.

A number of different types of oncogenes have been identified. They all have harmless counterparts in normal genes which have not been perverted by viral action. It is believed that a few common human cancers, such as liver, cervical and penile cancer, are caused by viruses, but this has been thought not to apply to most other cancers. Research work on oncogenes may prove this wrong.

There is also the possibility that the influence of radiation (as in UV rays) or of ingested chemicals can, in the same way as a virus, cause a gene to mutate and change its nature, with similar effects on the genes' signalling system.

Or it may be a case of missing instructions. This postulates the existence of cancer-suppressor genes, whose function is to prevent uncontrolled proliferation. Some genes instruct the undifferentiated cells of an embryo to grow and develop into a foetus; when the process is complete, another gene switches it off. But in the absence of the cancer-suppressor gene, the process can be switched on again, years later, by some physiological mischance, causing a tumour to start to grow. This is thought to be the mechanism in the case of one rare childhood cancer, retinoblastoma: if the cause of it is a missing gene, this could explain why this is an inheritable cancer. The fact that many types of tumour consist of undifferentiated, quasi-embryonic cells may confirm the supposition that some process that should have ceased in the course of foetal development, has been reactivated.

Possibly both explanations are valid: in some cancers the instructions have gone wrong, whilst in some others they simply are not there.

preventing cancer

If a way could be found of immunising people against all types of cancer, this could lead to the total elimination of the disease, just as smallpox has been eliminated. At present, this is only a distant hope: immunologists are trying to arrive at a fuller understanding of the body's immune system, by a study of lymphocytes, those white blood cells whose function it is to identify and destroy invaders. This, it is hoped, will eventually enable scientists to find a way of stimulating the lymphocytes to greater efficiency in ridding the body of invading viruses and tumour cells by 'recognising' them as foreign as soon as they appear and destroying them.

In the mean time, the World Health Organisation is conducting field trials with hepatitis B vaccine in several third world countries. This virus-caused disease is itself a cause of liver cancer, and it is hoped that the very effective vaccine will, by reducing the incidence of hepatitis B, also reduce the incidence of the cancer in the field trial areas. It will not be known for some years whether this hope is to be confirmed.

A vaccine has been experimentally made against the Epstein-Barr (EB) virus (which is associated with glandular fever and Burkitt's lymphoma) and may soon be used to immunise humans.

Another kind of prevention is being tried out in Britain with the help of volunteers: 2,000 healthy women in the high-risk group for breast cancer (those aged 50 to 70 and whose mother or sisters had the disease) will be given the anti-hormone drug tamoxifen for at least five years. They will be monitored to see whether this reduces the incidence of the disease among them. There will be a control group of another 2,000 women, receiving dummy pills, against whom the treated group can be checked. Tamoxifen is already widely used to suppress oestrogen production in women who have had breast cancer, and it is thought that it might also prevent the disease from starting.

early detection of cancer

Work is being done to find ways of detecting cancer in its earliest stages, when it is most curable, but also generally symptomless. In the USA, instruments are being developed that are sensitive enough to measure the minute amounts of microwave radiation emitted by the human body. The fact that tumour tissue emits different amounts of radiation from healthy tissue could lead to the development of a new diagnostic technique.

Gene probes are being developed, in the USA and elsewhere, to test for the presence of some inheritable diseases. The probes are strands of DNA carrying the gene that transmits the disease, and they are used to test for the presence of the same gene in the tissues of the unborn foetus. This technique may prove adaptable for testing for the genes of certain inheritable cancers.

advances in cancer therapy

Improved ways of treating cancer are being sought in surgery, radiotherapy, and, particularly in chemotherapy.

radiotherapy

Neutrons are said to be better than X-rays at killing hypoxic tumour cells, that is those which are able to flourish with a very low oxygen supply. As an alternative, drugs which make hypoxic cells more sensitive to X-rays are being used experimentally. However, it is necessary for clinical trials now being undertaken in Britain to confirm that these new methods have some clear advantages over standard X-ray therapy before their routine use would be considered justified.

hyperbaric oxygen therapy
The other way of destroying hypoxic cancer cells is by increasing the supply of oxygen to them. This can be achieved by placing the patient in an enclosure and filling it with oxygen under high pressure during the exposure to the X-rays.

chemotherapy

The biggest problem of cytotoxic drugs – their inability to discriminate between diseased and healthy tissue – may be on the way to being solved. There are a number of new drugs on trial (though progress here is rather slow). Many of these are analogues of existing drugs, that is, of the same basic structure but modified by biochemists. These drugs are often as effective – but less toxic, and so produce less severe side-effects.

monoclonal antibodies

An antibody is a protein produced by the immune system in response to the presence of an invading antigen (that is, a foreign substance such as a bacterium or virus). The antibody combines with the antigen and neutralises it. An antibody is specific: like a key that will fit only its own lock, an antibody will fit only on its corresponding antigen, ignoring others, and this feature is proving most useful.

Cell fusion techniques have made it possible to grow, under laboratory conditions, generations of cells that produce antibodies which identify and home in on antigens on the surface of particular cancer cells. These are called monoclonal antibodies, because they are clones – identical copies – of one particular antibody. Each kind of cancer cell has its own antigens, and it should be possible to produce a monoclonal antibody for each of these.

The happy prospect that this opens up is that of coupling monoclonal antibodies with some cytotoxic drugs, and injecting this combination into the tumour site, in the certainty that the antibodies will unite only with the appropriate tumour-cell antigens, so delivering the drug directly to the target, and sparing the healthy cells. When a tumour produces several antigens, a combination of several monoclonals could be used to deliver the drug.

This accurate targeting would mean that much more potent cytotoxic drugs could be used than is at present possible: for instance, ricin, a deadly toxin, which, given systemically in the conventional way, would kill patient and tumour together. Monoclonal antibodies could be used most effectively following cancer surgery, to kill remaining tumour tissue and any secondary tumours.

Treatment with monoclonal antibodies is not yet available and is still at an experimental stage. It may or may not prove practicable. If clinical trials confirm the usefulness of the technique, however, it could completely transform the prospects for chemotherapy – but this will not be known for some years yet.

Monoclonal antibodies are also being tried out as aids to radiotherapy. Tagged with radioactive isotopes, they make it easier to assess the extent of a tumour.

The possibility of using monoclonal antibodies to concentrate cytotoxic drugs on tumour areas has stimulated the search for more effective drugs, since side-effects from damage to healthy cells should no longer be a major problem.

biological response modification

Much research is being devoted to 'natural' drugs, derived from proteins that occur naturally in human tissues, and which are part of the armoury of the immune system. These drugs work rather differently from cytotoxic drugs. Although they also destroy cancer cells, they are less apt to devastate the normal ones. In some cases, they are anti-viral agents, and their effectiveness may be related to this; in other cases, the drugs are said to operate as differentiation modifiers, causing the immature undifferentiated cancer cells to assume a mature, differentiated form and the non-invasive behaviour that goes with this.

interferon

This is a protein naturally produced by the body in response to virus attack. At present it is found in three forms: alpha, beta and gamma, each form derived from different cells of the immune system. Originally, interferon had to be isolated from actual human blood cells, but now, thanks to genetic engineering techniques, it can be grown in bacteria, outside the body.

Wild claims, that it was a cancer cure-all were once made for interferon, and it has not lived up to them. However, alpha interferon has proved effective against a rare type of cancer, hairy-cell leukaemia, and there seems a good chance that the interferons will prove useful in treating cancers of those tissues from which they are derived. For instance, it seems that beta interferon, produced from epithelial (lining) cells, may prove effective in treating cancers of these tissues.

lymphotoxin

This is also a protein: it is manufactured by the white blood cells and, like interferon, occurs naturally in minute amounts only, but is now being produced in usable amounts by genetically converted E. Coli bacteria. Lymphotoxin is a tumour necrosis factor (TNF): it has the ability to kill cancer cells. It is believed to work by encouraging the production of other anti-cancer agents, such as interferons and macrophages, large cells whose function is to clear up foreign substances.

Interleukin-2

This, too, will probably not turn out to be a panacea, though it has unwisely been greeted as one. It is yet another attempt to bolster up the potency of the immune system, and is still only in the early trial stages. Interleukin-2 (IL-2) is a natural protein: a growth factor which stimulates the multiplication of the patient's own healthy white blood cells. These cells are taken from the patient, treated with IL-2 and returned to him, plus an additional dose of IL-2. This is systemic therapy, working on the whole body, and it is hoped that it will provide a way of treating disseminated cancer without the distressing side-effects of cytotoxic drugs. However, the treatment has been found to have side-effects of its own, notably fluid retention, which can lead to kidney, liver and respiratory problems. It is too soon to say whether IL-2 will justify the hopes invested in it.

cutting a tumour's lifeline

There is another kind of approach that uses a natural protein: one that hopes to turn cancer's own weapons against itself. Like all tissues, tumours need a blood supply to survive, and they are able to rig up their own supply lines: as a tumour grows, neighbouring blood vessels sprout capillaries, tiny blood vessels, to feed it. This process is called angiogenesis. Its origin has been traced to a protein found in human cancer cells. This protein has been isolated and named angiogenin. It opens up new possibilities: if a tumour could be deprived of angiogenin, it should (in theory) lose its blood supply and wither away. Whether this will work in practice – since other factors beside angiogenin contribute to the growth of blood vessels – remains to be seen.

natural drugs?

Many scientists believe that the future of therapy lies with 'natural' drugs (yet to be discovered) which will, instead of killing tumour cells, encourage them to grow up and start behaving normally. This hope depends on the theory that some cancer cells are Peter Pan cells, arrested at an embryonic stage of development. Research is being done on ways to start them specialising and maturing. It is too early to say whether this approach will yield results.

other new treatments

Hardly a month passes without success being reported in some part of the world for a new cancer therapy: delivering electric current to a tumour (Sweden); using rayon fibre filters to extract cancer-encouraging agents from the blood (Japan); using sound waves to keep cancer cells from multiplying (usa); and many more. The national press picks up news of such experimental work from scientific journals, and goes on to report them in terms which suggest that victory over cancer is just around the corner. But closer reading shows that things are not nearly so advanced: the work is only in its earlier experimental stages. Years pass, and nothing more is heard: presumably the new treatment did not come up to scratch, but few newspapers will bother to report that.

Cancer research, like any other research, is a catalogue in which lost hopes greatly outnumber the viable ones, but there are now quite a few of the latter.

Eminent researchers are fond of announcing that cancer will be done away with 'in our lifetime'. Realists may note that this will not happen in the lifetime of many cancer sufferers alive today. Neverthess, things do seem to be looking up, as cancer therapy moves away from its limited repertoire of surgery, chemotherapy and radiotherapy, in search of treatments at once more reliable and less devastating.

If the treatment of cancer maintains the progress it has made in the last forty years, the outlook should be considerably more and more hopeful. The five-year survival rate for all cancer patients has gone up steadily:

5-year survival – all cancer patients

Year		%
1900	less than	5
1949		25
1968		33
1978		42
1985		50

The outlook for some individual cancers is still more hopeful; some are now considered almost 100% curable. A radical decrease in smoking would do as much for cancer statistics as the treatments now under trial – lung cancer is one of the hardest to treat and is also one of the most preventable.

SOME ORGANISATIONS

There exists numerous organisations concerned with cancer. Some of them were founded to help sufferers from cancer in various ways: they may offer moral support through contact with fellow-sufferers, or nursing facilities, or special care for terminal patients, or advice on coping with problems that may arise from cancer treatment. Other organisations are there to further the cause of cancer research: some of these actually carry out research, while the others raise funds for this purpose. Still other organisations are concerned with the prevention of cancer, and aim to educate the public in this respect. Some of the bodies listed here belong to more than one category: for example, they may both offer help and seek to raise funds.

Many of them are charitable associations, some are staffed by volunteers who work from their own homes, so the addresses given here may change, as one voluntary worker takes over from another. There is usually a shortage of funds, so a stamped self-addressed envelope should be enclosed with written enquiries – and a donation is generally welcome.

self-help and support groups

BACUP **(British Association of Cancer United Patients)**
121/123 Charterhouse Square
London EC1M 6AA
telephone: 01-608 1661

Dr. Vicky Clement-Jones

Battersea Cancer Support Group
London Production Centre
Broomhill Road
Wandsworth
London SW18 4JQ
telephone: 01-871 3586

Roger Potter

C.A.L.L. **(Cancer Aid and Listening Line)**
49 Clothorn Road
Didsbury, Manchester
telephone: 061-445 0754

secretary: Anne Eardley

Cancer Contact
Mercers
High Street
Cuckfield
Sussex RH17 5JU
telephone: 0444-454043

founder and organiser: Ms Kit Mouat

Cancerlink
46A Pentonville Road
London N1 9HF
telephone: 01-833 2451

information officer: Amanda Kelsey
  S.R.N., S.C.M.

C.A.R.E. **(Cancer Aftercare and**
  Rehabilitation Society)
Lodge Cottage
Timsbury
Bath BA3 1LF
telephone: 0761-70731

secretary: G. W. Poole

help for post-surgery patients

Colostomy Welfare Group
38–39 Eccleston Square
London SW1V 1PB
telephone: 01-828 5175

welfare officer: Mrs. Catherine
Richards

Ileostomy Association of Great
  Britain and Ireland
Amblehurst House
Chobham
Woking
Surrey
GU24 8PZ
telephone: 09905-8277

Mastectomy Association
26 Harrison Street
Kings Cross
London WC1H 8JG
telephone: 01-837 0908

administrator: Mrs. S. A. Legge

National Association of
  Laryngectomee Clubs
Fourth Floor
39 Eccleston Square
London SW1V 1PB
telephone: 01-834 2857

Sexual and Personal
  Relationships of the Disabled
286 Camden Road
London N7 0BJ
telephone: 01-607 8851/2

education and training officer:
  Dr. Mary Davies

Stoma Advisory Service
Abbot Laboratories Ltd.
Queenborough
Kent
ME11 5EL
telephone: 0795-663371

divisional manager, patient care
  division: T. K. Cottam

Urostomy Association (formerly
  Urinary Conduit Association)
8 Coniston Close
Dane Bank
Denton
Manchester M34 2EW
telephone: 061-336 8818

Mrs. V. Kings

homeopathic medicine

**The British Homeopathic
  Association**
27A Devonshire Street
London W1N 1RJ
telephone: 01-935 2163

**Homeopathic Development
  Foundation Ltd**
19a Cavendish Square
London W1M 9AD
telephone: 01-629 3205

**Royal London Homeopathic
  Hospital**
Great Ormond Street
London WC1N 3HR
telephone: 01-837 8833

complementary and alternative treatments

ANAC **(Association for New
  Approaches to Cancer)**
c/o The Seekers Trust
Addington Park
Maidstone
Kent
ME19 5BL
telephone: 0732-848336

director: Donald Stevens

**Association for Therapeutic
  Healers**
Flat 51
67/69 Chancery Lane
London WC1
telephone: 01-831 9377

**Association of Hypnotists and
  Psychotherapists**
25 Market Square
Nelson
Lancashire
BB9 7LP
telephone: 0282-699378

Bristol Cancer Help Centre
see Cancer Help Centre (Bristol)

**British Holistic Medical
  Association**
179 Gloucester Place
London NW1 6DX
telephone: 01-262 5299

informationi officer: Mrs. Mary Toase

Cancer Help Centre (Bristol)
Grove House
Cornwallis Grove
Clifton
Bristol BS8 4PG
telephone: 0272-743216

Centre for Attitudinal Healing
P.O. Box 638
London SW3 4LN
telephone: 01-235 6733

secretary: Monica L. Askey

**Churches Council for Health and
   Healing**
St. Marylebone Parish Church
Marylebone Road
London NW1 5LT
telephone: 01-486 9644

**Confederation of Healing
   Organisations**
113 Hampstead Way
London NW11 7JN
telephone: 01-455 2638

chairman: Denis L. Haviland

**Gerson Nutritional Cancer
   Therapy**
c/o Ann Archer
31 Ranmoor Gardens
Harrow
Middlesex HA1 1UQ
telephone: 01-427 0060
or: *Margaret Straus*
   (Dr. Gerson's granddaughter)
Via Nazionale 87
22050 – Colico (CO)
Italy

Guild of Health Ltd.
26 Queen Anne Street
London W1M 9LB
telephone: 01-580 2492

**Institute for Complementary
   Medicine**
21 Portland Place
London WC1N 3AF
telephone: 01-636 9543

**Matthew Manning Centre
   (Healing)**
39 Abbeygate Street
Bury St. Edmunds
Suffolk
IP33 1LW
telephone: 0284-69502

secretary: Miss Laura Webber

**National Federation of Spiritual
   Healers**
Old Manor Farm Studio
Church Street
Sunbury-on-Thames
Middlesex
W16 6RG
telephone: 09327- 83164

cancer prevention and education

**ASH (Action on Smoking and
   Health)**
5–11 Mortimer Street
London W1N 7RH
telephone: 01-637 9843

*hon. secretaries: Dr. Noel Olsen,
   and Dr. Muir Gray*

British Digestive Foundation
Room D
7 Chandos Street
Cavendish Square
London W1A 2LN
telephone: 01-580 1155

*executive secretary: Miss Joan
   Stuart*

Cancer Prevention Research Trust
36 Roehampton Vale
London SW15 3RY
telephone: 01-789 1262

V. M. Fellas

Cancer Prevention Society
Volunteer Centre
25 Wellington Street
Glasgow G2 6JJ
telephone: 041-226 4626

information assistant:
Vincent Turnbull

Dr. Jan De Winter Clinic for Cancer Prevention Advice
6 New Road
Brighton
telephone: 0273-727213

Manchester Regional Committee for Cancer Education
Kinnaird Road
Manchester M20 9QL
telephone: 061-434 7721

executive director: R. L. Davison

SPAID (Society for the Prevention of Asbestosis and Industrial Diseases)
38 Drapers Road
Enfield
Middlesex EN2 8LU
telephone: 01-366 1640

secretary: Nancy Tait

nursing and terminal care

Association of carers
Medway Homes
Balfour Road
Rochester
Kent ME4 6QU
telephone: 0634-813981/2

Hospice Information Service
St. Christopher's Hospice
Lawrie Park Road
Sydenham
London SE26 6DZ
telephone: 01-778 1240

Intractable Pain Society
Pain Relief Clinic
Basingstoke District Hospital
Aldermaston Road
Basingstoke
Hampshire RG24 9NA
telephone: 0256-52333

hon. secretary: Dr. Tim P. Nash.

Marie Curie Memorial Foundation
28 Belgrave Square
London SW1X 8QG
telephone: 01-235 3325

executive secretary: P. A. Sturgess

Macmillan Cancer Relief Fund
see National Society for Cancer
   Relief

**Malcolm Sargent Cancer Fund
   for Children**
14 Abingdon Road
London W8 6AF
telephone: 01-937 4548

general administrator: Sylvia Darley

National Society for Cancer Relief
(Macmillan Cancer Relief Fund)
Michael Sobell House
30 Dorset Square
London NW1 6QL
telephone: 01-402 8125

general secretary: S. H. Creswell

Sue Ryder Foundation
Cavendish
Sudbury
Suffolk
CO10 8AY
telephone: 0787-280252

Lady Ryder of Warsaw, C.M.G., O.B.E.

cancer research associations and fund-raising bodies

**Association for International
   Cancer Research**
Cancer Research Laboratory
Department of Chemistry
University of St. Andrews
Fife KY16 9ST
telephone: 0332 76161

director: Dr. Colin Thomson.

Cancer Research Campaign
2 Carlton House Terrace
London SW1Y 5AR
telephone: 01-930 8972

*cancer information officer:
   Miss E. D. Skinner*

Imperial Cancer Research Fund
P.O. Box No. 123
Lincoln's Inn Fields
London WC2A 3PX
telephone: 01-242 0200

secretary: A. B. L. Clarke C.B.E.

**Institute of Cancer Research and
   the Royal Marsden Hospital**
Clinical Academic Unit
Royal Marsden Hospital
Downs Road
Sutton
Surrey SM2 5PT
telephone: 01-642 6011

National Foundation for Cancer Research
7315 Wisconsin Avenue
Suite 332W
Bethesda
Maryland 20814
USA

Quest for a Test for Cancer
Woodbury
Harlow Road
Roydon
Essex CM19 5HF
telephone: 027979-2233

South Wales Research Council
Velindre Hospital
Whitchurch
Cardiff CF4 7XL
telephone: 0222-615888

hon. secretary: S. C. Walters.

Wessex Cancer Research Trust
Royal South Hampshire Hospital
Graham Road
Southampton SO9 4PE
telephone: 0703-29653

fund-raising and support groups for particular forms of cancer

CLIC **(The Cancer and Leukaemia in Childhood Trust)**
Pembroke House
11–12 Fremantle Square
Cotham
Bristol BS6 5TL
telephone: 0272-48844

secretary: Mrs. Gail Banham

Jeannie Campbell Breast Cancer Radiotherapy Appeal
29 St. Luke's Avenue
Ramsgate
Kent CT11 7JZ
telephone: 0843-596732/593193

chairman: Mr. Peter Hawkins

Kingston Trust
The Drove
Kempshott
Basingstoke
Hampshire RG22 5LU
telephone: 0256-52320

Leukaemia Research Fund
43 Great Ormond Street
London WC1N 3JJ
telephone: 01-405 0101

D. L. Osborne

Leukaemia Society
P.O. Box 82
Exeter
Devon EX2 5DP
telephone: 0392-218514

Neuroblastoma Society
"Woodlands"
Ordsall Park Road
Retford
Nottinghamshire DN22 7PJ
telephone: 07777-709238

Mrs. Janet Oldridge

Women's Health Information Centre
Ufton Centre
12 Ufton Road
London N1 5BY
telephone: 01-254 9094

Ms. Lisa Saffron

Womens National Cancer Control Campaign
1 South Audley Street
London W1Y 5DQ
telephone: 01-499 7532/4

director: Mrs. Alice Burns

GLOSSARY

adenoma
tumour of a gland

adjuvant
treatment (such as chemotherapy or radiotherapy) given to prevent the recurrence of a surgically removed tumour

adrenal glands
pair of endocrine glands situated above the kidneys and secreting adrenaline, hydrocortisone and other hormones

allopathic
medical practice of treating a disease with remedies whose effects are different from the symptoms of the disease (i.e. most conventional medicine), as against homeopathic

alpha-tocopherol
vitamin E

analgesic
drug to relieve pain

anaplastic (or undifferentiated)
the immature, embryonic appearance of many kinds of cancer cells
see also differentiation

androgen
a male sex hormone, for example, testosterone

anorexia
loss of appetite

antibody
a protein formed by lymphocytes in response to the presence of an antigen

antigen
a protein which is recognised by the immune system as 'non-self' and stimulates the production of antibodies

ascites
swelling of the abdomen, resembling pregnancy and resulting from a build-up of fluid

ascorbic acid
vitamin C

bacterium
a micro-organism which may serve as the agent of infection

basal cell carcinoma (or rodent ulcer)
a type of skin cancer, locally invasive but which seldom or never metastasises, thought to be caused by UV radiation in sunlight
see also malignant melanoma; squamous cell carcinoma

benign
non-cancerous; term for conglomerations of cells which grow in some tissues but do not invade or infiltrate other tissues
see also neoplasm; tumour

beta-carotene
yellow pigment found in many dark green and yellow vegetables and fruits, and converted by the body to retinol

biopsy
a test for detecting the presence of a malignant tumour, in which a specimen of the suspect tissue is removed for laboratory examination

carcinogenesis
the formation of a cancer

carcinoma
the group name for cancers originating in the epithelial tissues: the commonest type of cancer

cell
the basic unit from which all the tissues of the body are built up:

in the earliest stages of an embryo, cells are undifferentiated or unspecialised; as the embryo grows, they become differentiated and turn into specialised organs and tissues

cell membrane
a thin wall which separates each cell from other cells
see also nucleus; cytoplasm

cervix
neck; often used as abbreviation of cervix uteri, neck of the womb

chromosomes
structures made of DNA, 23 pairs of which exist in the nucleus of each cell, and containing all the genetic material for the cell to function. When the cell divides, the chromosomes duplicate and then divide so that each daughter cell gets a complete set (sex cells are different in having only 23 chromosomes, not 23 pairs);
see also gene

CT scanning
computer axial tomography: a refinement of X-ray investigation for the diagnosis of cancer

cyst
a swelling filled with fluid

cytology
the study of cells

cytoplasm
that part of a cell's protoplasm which is neither nucleus nor membrane

cytotoxic
literally, cell-poisoning: used of drugs and treatments which destroy tumour cells and also some healthy ones

differentiation
the changes that take place in the cells of an embryo, resulting in the development of different organs and tissues with specialised functions

DNA
abbreviation of deoxyribonucleic acid, the material of inheritance, present in the nucleus of every cell in the form of a double-stranded, helically-twisted chain
see also RNA

ductless glands
see endocrine glands

embryo
in human beings, unborn child's earliest stage of development, during the eight weeks (approximately) following conception; after this, it is called a foetus

endocrine glands (or ductless glands)
glands which release hormones directly into the bloodstream, to circulate around the body; some organs, such as the ovaries, the testes and the pancreas, also function as endocrine glands

endometrium
the lining of the womb (uterus)

endoscope
an optical instrument equipped with a light, for examining the insides of hollow organs. It comes in various forms: gastroscope for the stomach, cystoscope for the bladder, sigmoidoscope and colonoscope for the large bowel, colposcope for the cervix uteri, bronchoscope for the lungs

enzyme
protein which activates chemical reactions in a cell while itself remaining unchanged

epidemiology
the study of the incidence and patterns of diseases in populations

epithelium
layers of cells which cover the outside of organs (e.g. skin), or line the inside, (e.g. bowel lining or stomach lining)

ethanol
ethyl alcohol; pure alcohol

flora (colonic)
micro-organisms living in the healthy bowel, and involved in breaking down food residue

foetus
name for the unborn child in the second stage of growth: from about eight weeks after conception, until it is fully developed
see also embryo

gene
a hereditary factor; one of the units of which chromosomes are composed: each gene is responsible for some characteristic which is passed on when a cell divides to reproduce

haematologist
medical specialist concerned with diseases of the blood

haemoglobin
the red pigment which gives red blood cells their colour; it transports oxygen from the lungs to the tissues of the body

hepatoma
cancer of the liver

Hodgkin's disease
a lymphoma of the lymph nodes and spleen

homeopathic
the practice of treating disease with minute amounts of substances which, if given at full strength, would produce the same symptoms as the disease, on the principle of 'like cures like'
see also allopathic

hormone
a chemical substance secreted into the bloodstream by one of the endocrine glands, to influence the development and functioning of other organs

involution
gradual reduction, shrinkage

ionising radiations
electromagnetic waves and particles which carry enough energy to alter the normal configuration of atoms and molecules through which they pass, thus changing the properties of tissue penetrated by them, usually resulting in damage

isotope
a variant form of an element; the atoms of the different isotopes of the same element have the same number of protons but different numbers of neutrons. Some isotopes of an element may be radioactive, that is, emit high-energy electrons (beta-rays) or heavier particles (alpha-particles) as well as electromagnetic radiation

Kaposi's sarcoma
a form of skin cancer rare in itself which, however, is the common result of the collapse of the body's immune system following infection with HTLV-III, the AIDS virus

laetrile
a non-orthodox cancer remedy (forms of which are also called amygdalin, nitriloside or vitamin B17) derived from bitter almonds or cherry and apricot kernels

leukaemia
the group name for cancers affecting the white blood cells and the bone marrow in which they are produced

local
used of treatments, e.g. radiotherapy, which are concentrated on particular areas of the body

localised
the term for a cancer which has not spread beyond the organ in which it originated

lumpectomy
a surgical procedure for breast tumours, in which the tumour is removed, with some surrounding tissue, but the whole breast is not removed
see also mastectomy

lymph
a yellowish fluid, derived from blood, which circulates round the body, draining the tissues of impurities such as bacteria

lymphatic system
a system of vessels (rather like blood vessels) which drains lymph, a blood derivative, from spaces between the cells, and transports it through all parts of the body (except the central nervous system), finally returning it to the blood circulation. At various points in the network, lymph nodes act as filtering stations, removing bacteria and other foreign matter

lymph nodes (or lymph glands)
filtering points in the lymphatic system. They are classified according to their sites: for example cervical (neck), axillary (armpit), mediastinal (chest), abdominal (belly), inguinal (groin)

lymphocytes
a type of white blood cell, whose task is to maintain the body's immunity to infection by forming antibodies; they include T-cells, B-cells and NK-cells

lymphoma
the group name for cancers of the lymphatic system

malignant
cancerous; term for conglomerations of cells which show a tendency to infiltrate or invade tissues to which they do not belong
see also neoplasm; tumour; metastasis

malignant melanoma
a type of skin cancer arising from pigment cells usually in the skin, sometimes in eye or mucosae (mouth, anus and genital); it

may arise in a previous mole or as a new lesion, sometimes associated with sun exposure or sunburn; it may metastasise

mammography
a method of examining the breast with the help of X-rays

mastectomy
the surgical procedure for breast cancer in which the whole breast is removed; sometimes the adjacent lymph nodes are also removed

melanin
brown pigment present to a greater or lesser extent in the skin, hair and eyes (the iris) of all human beings except albinos

melanoma
see malignant melanoma

membrane
see cell membrane

menarche
the start of menstruation

mesothelioma
a cancer of the membrane which lines the lungs, the chest cavity and the abdominal cavity: generally attributed to exposure to asbestos

metastasis
the ability of malignant tumours to infiltrate tissues distant from those in which they originated, by dispersing cancer cells through the blood circulation or the lymphatic system

mitosis
a process in which a cell reproduces itself by dividing, to produce two daughter cells identical in every respect to the parent cell. The process begins with the DNA in the nucleus duplicating itself, so that when the cell divides, each daughter cell gets a complete set of chromosomes

mutation
an untoward alteration to cellular DNA which causes the production of abnormal cells

myelography
X-ray examination of the spinal cord

narcotic
a drug which numbs the sensation of pain by dulling consciousness

NMR
abbreviation of nuclear magnetic resonance scanning, an investigative method used in diagnosing cancer

neoplasm
literally, new form: a lump or growth of surplus cells; also called a tumour

nucleus
the controlling unit of a cell, having its own membrane, and containing coded instructions in the form of DNA, which tell the cell how to perform its functions and to replicate itself
see also chromosomes; genes

oestrogen
female sex hormone, thought to be implicated in cancer of the breast and the womb

oncogene
a gene capable of causing malignant changes in cells; thought to be originally a normal gene which has become perverted by the action of a virus or some other agency

oncologist
a cancer specialist

oophorectomy
surgical removal of the ovaries

orchidectomy
surgical removal of the testes

organelle
a structure in a cell which carries out a specialised function; it is to a cell what an organ is to a body

palpation
examining a patient by touching or feeling with the fingers

pituitary gland
endocrine gland, situated below the brain, which regulates the action of the other endocrine glands

placebo
a dummy remedy, without any active ingredients, commonly given to a control group of patients as an aid in assessing the effectiveness of drugs being tested on human subjects

platelets
small red blood cells playing an important part in clotting

polyposis coli
a hereditary condition in which tumours, called polyps, grow in the colon; they are benign but signal a pre-cancerous state

protein
organic compound which is essential to the existence of all living matter. Countless proteins exist, each being made up from different combinations of amino-acid molecules

protoplasm
the protein material of which all cells are composed
see also cytoplasm

pyelography
x-ray examination of kidneys

radiation
the emission of energy in the form of particles or electromagnetic waves, from sources which may be natural (e.g. sunlight) or man-made (e.g. x-rays)
see also ionising radiation; UV

radiotherapist
specialist who treats disease with ionising radiation

remission
the complete disappearance of symptoms for a time. In most types of cancer, if the symptoms have not returned after a given period, the patient is considererd cured

retinol
vitamin A

RNA
abbreviation of ribonucleic acid, present in the cell in the form of a chain corresponding to the DNA, whose instructions it passes on, acting as a template for the production of new proteins

sarcoma
the group name for cancers originating in bone, muscle and connective tissue

selenium
element present in trace amounts in many foods

squamous cell carcinoma
skin cancer, slow to spread and metastasise, thought to be caused by exposure to UV radiation in sunlight
see also basal cell carcinoma; malignant melanoma

systemic
used of treatments, such as chemotherapy, which affect the whole body, as against local treatment

thyroid gland
an endocrine gland situated in the neck, and secreting thyroxine and other hormones

tissues
the cell structures of which all parts or organs of the body are composed, each kind of tissue has a specialised function in the body

tumour
a mass of superfluous cells forming a lump, growth or swelling; also called a neoplasm. Tumours are malignant if they tend to invade other tissues, benign if they are non-invasive

UV
short for ultra-violet; a type of radiation occurring in sunlight and thought to be implicated in the formation of skin cancers

virus
an infective agent, consisting of a length of DNA or RNA enclosed in protein, and incapable of independent life; it lives and reproduces by invading a normal cell, on which it becomes parasitic.

MODDOR
953753
4.7.86